UNDERSTANDING RACIAL AND ETHNIC DIFFERENCES IN HEALTH IN LATE LIFE

A RESEARCH AGENDA

Panel on Race, Ethnicity, and Health in Later Life

Rodolfo A. Bulatao and Norman B. Anderson,
Editors

Committee on Population

Division of Behavioral and Social Sciences and Education

NATIONAL RESEARCH COUNCIL
OF THE NATIONAL ACADEMIES

D1400557

THE NATIONAL ACADEMIES PRESS
Washington, D.C.
www.nap.edu

THE NATIONAL ACADEMIES PRESS • 500 Fifth Street, N.W. • Washington, D.C. 20001

NOTICE: The project that is the subject of this report was approved by the Governing Board of the National Research Council, whose members are drawn from the councils of the National Academy of Sciences, the National Academy of Engineering, and the Institute of Medicine. The members of the committee responsible for the report were chosen for their special competences and with regard for appropriate balance.

This study was supported by Contract No. N01-OD-4-2139, TO #71 between the National Academies and the National Institute of Aging and by a grant from the Andrew W. Mellon Foundation. Any opinions, findings, conclusions, or recommendations expressed in this publication are those of the authors and do not necessarily reflect the views of the organizations or agencies that provided support for the project.

Library of Congress Cataloging-in-Publication Data

Understanding racial and ethnic differences in health in late life : a research agenda / Panel on Race, Ethnicity, and Health in Later Life, Committee on Population, Division of Behavioral and Social Sciences and Education ; Rodolfo A. Bulatao and Norman B. Anderson, editors.

    p. ; cm.

"This volume is the Panel's final report. The workshop papers are available in a companion volume, Critical perspectives on racial and ethnic differences in health in late life"— Pref.

Updates work from: Racial and ethnic differences in the health of older Americans. 1997. Includes bibliographical references and index.

ISBN 0-309-09247-7 (pbk.)

1. Minorities—Health and hygiene—United States. 2. Ethnic groups—Health and hygiene—United States. 3. Older people—Health and hygiene—United States. 4. Health services accessibility—United States. 5. Discrimination in medical care—United States. 6. Health status indicators—United States. 7. Health and race—United States. 8. Social medicine—United States.

[DNLM: 1. Continental Population Groups—United States. 2. Geriatric Assessment—United States. 3. Ethnic Groups—United States. 4. Health Services Accessibility—Aged—United States. 5. Socioeconomic Factors—Aged—United States. WT 30 U45 2004] I. Bulatao, Rodolfo A., 1944- II. Anderson, Norman B. III. National Research Council (U.S.). Panel on Race, Ethnicity, and Health in Later Life. IV. Racial and ethnic differences in the health of older Americans.

RA448.4.U52 2004
362.1'089'00973—dc22

2004016831

Additional copies of this report are available from the National Academies Press, 500 Fifth Street, N.W., Lockbox 285, Washington, D.C. 20055; (800) 624-6242 or (202) 334-3313 (in the Washington metropolitan area); http://www.nap.edu.

Printed in the United States of America.

Suggested citation: National Research Council. (2004). *Understanding Racial and Ethnic Differences in Health in Late Life: A Research Agenda*. Panel on Race, Ethnicity, and Health in Later Life. Roldolfo A. Bulatao and Norman B. Anderson, editors. Committee on Population, Division of Behavioral and Social Sciences and Education. Washington, DC: The National Academies Press.

THE NATIONAL ACADEMIES
Advisers to the Nation on Science, Engineering, and Medicine

The **National Academy of Sciences** is a private, nonprofit, self-perpetuating society of distinguished scholars engaged in scientific and engineering research, dedicated to the furtherance of science and technology and to their use for the general welfare. Upon the authority of the charter granted to it by the Congress in 1863, the Academy has a mandate that requires it to advise the federal government on scientific and technical matters. Dr. Bruce M. Alberts is president of the National Academy of Sciences.

The **National Academy of Engineering** was established in 1964, under the charter of the National Academy of Sciences, as a parallel organization of outstanding engineers. It is autonomous in its administration and in the selection of its members, sharing with the National Academy of Sciences the responsibility for advising the federal government. The National Academy of Engineering also sponsors engineering programs aimed at meeting national needs, encourages education and research, and recognizes the superior achievements of engineers. Dr. Wm. A. Wulf is president of the National Academy of Engineering.

The **Institute of Medicine** was established in 1970 by the National Academy of Sciences to secure the services of eminent members of appropriate professions in the examination of policy matters pertaining to the health of the public. The Institute acts under the responsibility given to the National Academy of Sciences by its congressional charter to be an adviser to the federal government and, upon its own initiative, to identify issues of medical care, research, and education. Dr. Harvey V. Fineberg is president of the Institute of Medicine.

The **National Research Council** was organized by the National Academy of Sciences in 1916 to associate the broad community of science and technology with the Academy's purposes of furthering knowledge and advising the federal government. Functioning in accordance with general policies determined by the Academy, the Council has become the principal operating agency of both the National Academy of Sciences and the National Academy of Engineering in providing services to the government, the public, and the scientific and engineering communities. The Council is administered jointly by both Academies and the Institute of Medicine. Dr. Bruce M. Alberts and Dr. Wm. A. Wulf are chair and vice chair, respectively, of the National Research Council.

www.national-academies.org

PANEL ON RACE, ETHNICITY, AND HEALTH IN LATER LIFE

NORMAN B. ANDERSON (*Chair*), American Psychological Association, Washington, DC
EILEEN M. CRIMMINS, Andrus Gerontology Center, University of Southern California
ANGUS S. DEATON,* Woodrow Wilson School of Public and International Affairs, Princeton University
DAVID V. ESPINO, Department of Family and Community Medicine, University of Texas Health Science Center, San Antonio
JAMES S. HOUSE, Institute of Gerontology, University of Michigan Ann Arbor
JAMES S. JACKSON, Department of Psychology, University of Michigan Ann Arbor
CHRISTOPHER JENCKS, John F. Kennedy School of Government, Harvard University
GERALD E. MCCLEARN, Center for Developmental and Health Genetics, Pennsylvania State University
ALBERTO PALLONI, Department of Sociology, University of Wisconsin–Madison
TERESA E. SEEMAN, School of Medicine, University of California, Los Angeles
JAMES P. SMITH, RAND Corporation, Santa Monica, CA
EUGENIA Y.-H. WANG, School of Medicine, University of Louisville
DAVID R. WILLIAMS, Department of Sociology, University of Michigan Ann Arbor

RODOLFO A. BULATAO, *Study Director*
BARNEY COHEN, *Director, Committee on Population*
BANGHWA LEE CASADO, *Research Intern*
CHRISTINE COVINGTON CHEN, *Senior Program Assistant*
ANTHONY S. MANN, *Senior Program Assistant*

*Until October 2002.

Preface

The Panel on Race, Ethnicity, and Health in Later Life was established in 2001 under the auspices of the Committee on Population of the National Research Council (NRC). The panel's task was to inform the National Institute on Aging about recent research findings on racial and ethnic disparities in later life and to help in developing a future research agenda for reducing them. This project was a follow-up to a 1994 Committee on Population workshop, which resulted in a volume of papers published by the National Academy Press, *Racial and Ethnic Differences in the Health of Older Americans.*

The panel was asked, first to organize a 2-day workshop bringing together leading researchers from a variety of disciplines and professional orientations to summarize current research and to identify research priorities. That workshop was held in March 2002 in Washington, DC. The panel was also asked to produce a summary of the state of knowledge, based on the workshop, and to provide recommendations for further work. The initial plan called for the papers and the panel report to be published in a single volume, but ultimately it was decided to publish the papers and the panel report separately. This volume is the panel's final report. The workshop papers are available in a companion volume, *Critical Perspectives on Racial and Ethnic Differences in Health in Late Life.*

The panel benefited greatly from the workshop papers and thanks the following individuals for their contribution to the workshop and the resulting volume: Gary D. Sandefur, Mary E. Campbell, Jennifer Eggerling-Boeck, Robert A. Hummer, Maureen R. Benjamins, Richard G. Rogers, Jennifer J.

Manly, Richard Mayeux, Clyde Hertzman, Alberto Palloni, Douglas Ewbank, Guillermina Jasso, Douglas S. Massey, Mark E. Rosenzweig, James P. Smith, Richard S. Cooper, Eileen M. Crimmins, Mark D. Hayward, Teresa E. Seeman, Carlos Mendes de Leon, Thomas A. Glass, Jeffrey D. Morenoff, John Lynch, Marilyn A. Winkleby, Catherine Cubbin, Hector F. Myers, Wei-Chin Hwang, Rodney Clark, Julian F. Thayer, Bruce H. Friedman, Amitabh Chandra, Jonathan S. Skinner, David M. Cutler, James Y. Nazroo, Debbie Bradshaw, Rosana Norman, Ria Laubscher, Michelle Schneider, Nolwazi Mbananga, and Krisela Steyn.

The panel met multiple times over the course of the project to plan and hold the workshop and to digest and interpret the presentations. This report reflects the intense deliberations of the full panel, based on the papers and the members' own expertise.

This report has been reviewed in draft form by individuals chosen for their diverse perspectives and technical expertise, in accordance with procedures approved by the NRC's Report Review Committee. The purpose of this independent review is to provide candid and critical comments that will assist the institution in making its published report as sound as possible and to ensure that the report meets institutional standards for objectivity, evidence, and responsiveness to the study charge. The review comments and draft manuscript remain confidential to protect the integrity of the deliberative process. We thank the following individuals for their review of this report: Stuart H. Altman, National Health Policy, Heller Graduate School, Brandeis University; Lisa Berkman, School of Public Health, Harvard University; Janet Currie, Department of Economics, University of California, Los Angeles; Mark D. Hayward, Social Science Research Institute, Pennsylvania State University; Judith R. Lave, Health Policy and Management, Graduate School of Public Health, University of Pittsburgh; Spero Manson, American Indian and Alaska Native Programs, University of Colorado Health Sciences Center, Aurora, CO; Kyriakos S. Markides, Division of Sociomedical Sciences, Department of Preventive Medicine and Community Health, University of Texas Medical Branch, Galveston, TX; Thomas G. McGuire, Department of Health Care Policy, Harvard Medical School; Gary D. Sandefur, Department of Sociology, Institute of Poverty, University of Wisconsin–Madison; and Kenneth W. Wachter, Department of Demography, University of California, Berkeley.

Although the reviewers listed above have provided many constructive comments and suggestions, they were not asked to endorse the conclusions or recommendations nor did they see the final draft of the report before its release. The review of this report was overseen by Larry Bumpass, Center for Demography and Ecology, University of Wisconsin–Madison, and Harold C. Sox, Annals of Internal Medicine, American College of Physicians of Internal Medicine, Philadelphia, PA. Appointed by the NRC, they were responsible for making certain that an independent examination of this report was carried out in accordance with institutional procedures and that all review comments were carefully considered. Responsibility for the final content of this report rests entirely with the authoring committee and the institution.

The panel is grateful to the sponsors of the project, the National Institute of Aging and the Andrew W. Mellon Foundation. Besides providing funding, the representatives of these organizations were a valuable source of information and advice to the panel.

The panel was fortunate to have the services of the study director, Randy Bulatao, who worked closely with panel members to draft and edit the report. Barney Cohen, director of the Committee on Population, oversaw the work and managed the final stages of the process. Special thanks are due to Christine Covington Chen for her superb administrative and logistic support, to Eugenia Grohman for skillfully editing the manuscript, to Kirsten Sampson Snyder for navigating the report through review, and to Anthony Mann and Yvonne Wise for preparing the final manuscript for publication.

Norman B. Anderson, *Chair*
Panel on Race, Ethnicity, and Health in Later Life

Contents

Executive Summary

An enormous amount of research has confirmed the existence of large and persistent differences in health status between various racial and ethnic groups in the United States. Most of this research has focused on black-white differences: it consistently shows that despite rising life expectancy and general improvements in the health status of the U.S. population, blacks continue to experience significantly lower life expectancy than whites.

Over the last 20 years, research on these issues has largely shifted away from straightforward descriptive studies to attempts to identify the underlying determinants of the observed differences in health status by race as a step towards developing an integrated model of causal processes. Many different disciplines have made broad theoretical and empirical contributions to the debate, but, to date, scholars have not been able to integrate these diverse contributions into a unifying model of causal processes. Interdisciplinary dialogue in this area has sometimes been difficult. A major problem is that each discipline makes contributions that focus on their particular domains of interest, uses different underlying assumptions, and applies different standards of evidence when analyzing data. Thus, it is perhaps not surprising that after decades of research in this area, there are still large and persistent differences in health by racial and ethnic groups that have not been fully explained.

Making general statements about the importance of particular factors becomes much harder when racial and ethnic groups other than whites and blacks are included in the discussion. Although some minority older adults, particularly blacks and, generally, American Indians and Alaska Natives, are considerably less healthy than older whites, others, particularly Hispanics and Asians, are generally healthier. Yet these broad observations require qualifications: subgroups of each of these racial or ethnic groups vary in health status, and different indicators of health status also give different results. For example, age-adjusted mortality rates reinforce the general conclusions that Hispanics are healthier, on average, than whites, but from self-reported measures of health, Hispanics appear less healthy than whites.

Specific causes of death and specific morbidities lead to somewhat different rankings of racial and ethnic groups. For example, although blacks die more often than whites from most causes, their death rates from respiratory infections and pneumonia are lower than those for whites. Similarly, although Hispanics die less often than whites from most causes, they experience higher mortality from diabetes. Furthermore, looking across age groups, the contrasts are not consistent: most notably, the black disadvantage in old age is reversed at the oldest ages, when black mortality rates converge with those of whites and apparently fall below them.

Further complicating the study of racial and ethnic differences in health is the fluid nature of the social construct of race. Both academic and popular understandings of racial and ethnic identities have not been fixed and the picture of racial and ethnic differences in health has been heavily influenced by how these understandings have changed over time and how data on race and ethnicity have been collected.

To date, little of the research on racial and ethnic differences in health has been directed specifically towards the elderly, despite population projections that show that the population aged 65 and over is becoming increasingly diverse. Current projections suggest that, by 2050, while the total number of non-Hispanic whites aged 65 and over will double, the number of blacks aged 65 and over will more than triple, and the number of Hispanics will increase eleven-fold.

Recognizing the need for continuing research on racial and ethnic differences in health, as well as the increasing diversity of the U.S. population, the National Institutes of Aging asked the National Academies to (a) organize a 2-day workshop to bring together leading researchers from a variety of disciplines and professional orientations to summarize current research and to identify future direction for research in these areas and (b) to prepare a summary of the state of knowledge incorporating this information and providing recommendations for further work.

FINDINGS

Health differences involve a complexity of factors, including various processes of selection. Some racial and ethnic groups have high proportions of immigrants, some of whom are self-selected to be healthier than the native-born population. When older cohorts are compared, the groups reflect both selection from the original birth cohorts and differences in survival. Socioeconomic factors—education, income, wealth, occupational status, even residential neighborhood—are also important. Not only does low socioeconomic status impair health, but illness can in turn impose costs and reduce earnings and wealth. Yet the processes by which socioeconomic status affects health are not well understood. Furthermore, socioeconomic status is not always the dominant factor: for example, despite higher poverty rates, Hispanics have lower age-adjusted mortality rates than whites, and relatively low-income Vietnamese have lower mortality rates than relatively high-income Asian Indians.

Behavior risk factors—such as smoking, overeating, lack of exercise, and excessive alcohol use—clearly impair health, but their contribution to racial and ethnic differences is not always what one might expect. These risk factors are less common among Asians than whites (except for less exercise), which is consistent with better Asian health. However, they are more common among Hispanics than whites, despite lower Hispanic mortality. And because blacks generally smoke less than whites, this critical risk factor for several causes of death and illness serves to reduce differences between blacks and whites rather than increase them.

Cumulative prejudice and discrimination have been hypothesized to contribute to health differences among groups, but the processes by which they might do so are not well understood. Some evidence suggests that being discriminated against leads to psychological distress, with such negative health effects as elevated blood pressure, but not all studies support this finding.

Levels of stress, not only from experiencing discrimination but also from other pressures of life, are hypothesized to contribute to poor health, and they may vary across racial and ethnic groups. Models of the effects of stress on health such as allostatic load, cardiovascular reactivity, psycho-neuroimmunology, metabolic syndrome, and neurovisceral integration may have different predictive value among older persons of different racial and ethnic groups.

Differences in health care access and quality are well documented, and they may affect health, but how much of the racial and ethnic health differences may be accounted for by such differences in health care is unclear. Quality of health care varies geographically, and some of this variation may be related to the racial and ethnic composition of an area. Stereotypes held by providers have been hypothesized to be important, but the effects of such stereotypes on health differences in older ages is unclear. Patient compliance may account for some of the observed differences, and compliance varies by socioeconomic status, yet the patterns across racial and ethnic groups are not consistent.

The influence of each of these factors can cumulate over the life course, so that the health status of older cohorts reflects their entire life experiences. Research increasingly suggests that even early life experiences can contribute to late-life morbidity and age at mortality. Understanding health differences in old age therefore requires understanding influences across the life course.

Although deliberate interventions can affect individual health behaviors, interventions aimed at improving population health may exacerbate racial and ethnic differences, at least initially. For example, people with the most education and income may to be the first to quit smoking, lose weight, or start exercising in response to population-level interventions or when physicians recommend these changes, so that interventions targeted to particular groups may be needed to effect changes.

RESEARCH QUESTIONS AND NEEDS

Understanding the various factors that produce racial and ethnic group health differences in late life is important in the development of health policy. To date, what is known about the origins of racial and ethnic differences in health points in many directions, with findings coming from a variety of disciplines. And much of the research on particular determinants comes from work that does not focus specifically on older people. Consequently, researchers are still a long way from being able to construct a model that integrates all potential factors.

To advance the field, research is needed in each of the areas touched on above. The panel's list of research needs starts with the need to partition differences in morbidity and mortality in older populations to determine how much can be attributed to particular diseases or conditions and in turn how much of the differences in diseases and conditions can be assigned to major risk factors. Such analysis has been done to some extent for the general population, but not specifically for the elderly. If such partitioning can be accomplished, it should be possible to refine the research agenda to focus on the most critical areas. The list of research needs then focuses on verifying apparent health differences in cases where there are uncertainties, and on improving our understanding of the operation of and interaction among the major factors that contribute to racial and ethnic differences in health.

Three main themes underlie the panel's recommended research:

• The roots of health differences have to be examined across the life course, taking a longitudinal view and integrated account of the effects of such factors as socioeconomic status, behavior risk factors, and prejudice and discrimination, as well as the effects across cohorts and periods of selection processes and social policy.

• All factors should be investigated in terms of their links to stress and biopsychosocial mechanisms that lead to impaired health.

• Interventions designed to reduce health differences should be evaluated, along with determining the role of health care quality in racial and ethnic differences, which may range from possible geographic variability to differences in patient compliance and the use of alternative therapies.

Cutting across these themes is the need to investigate variability across and within multiple racial and ethnic groups.

The health disadvantages of a racial or ethnic group are a particular concern when that group is of low socioeconomic status or has experienced a history of prejudice or discrimination. Research is needed to identify the reasons for particular disadvantages and to understand mechanisms of influence. An additional challenge for public health is to achieve a balance between efforts to ameliorate racial and ethnic differences in health and efforts to improve population health in general. The panel recommends work on 18 research needs:

• Research Need 1: Attempt a systematic decomposition of racial and ethnic differences in mortality and morbidity among older people to determine the relative contribution of particular diseases or conditions. Try to assign differences in the prevalence of specific diseases and conditions to differences in the prevalence of major risk factors.

• Research Need 2: Clarify the contrasts between mortality rankings and morbidity rankings, particularly between older whites and Hispanics, and assess the relative contributions of diseases and conditions to differences in mortality and overall health.

• Research Need 3: When particular diseases are especially prevalent for specific racial and ethnic groups, collect more indicators of biological and functional performance in order to identify possibilities for intervention.

• Research Need 4: Identify and quantify the various selection processes that affect health differences among racial and ethnic groups.

• Research Need 5: Assess genetic and environmental factors in racial and ethnic differences in health simultaneously, in designs that permit identification of both main effects and interactions.

• Research Need 6: Clarify the degree to which socioeconomic status accounts for racial and ethnic differences in health outcomes over the life course.

• Research Need 7: Identify the mechanisms through which socioeconomic status produces racial and ethnic health differences in health among the elderly, and identify other factors that complicate its effects.

• Research Need 8: Study how behavior risk factors act over the life course in different racial and ethnic groups.

• Research Need 9: Characterize the distribution of social and psychological resources in different older populations and investigate whether their effects on health vary by race and ethnicity.
• Research Need 10: Determine the lifetime effects of prejudice and discrimination on health using longitudinal data and a framework that centers on stress and its effects.
• Research Need 11: Evaluate the effects of prejudice and discrimination on the health of minorities other than blacks.
• Research Need 12: Study populations of different racial and ethnic groups to assess the connection between health and the stresses that accumulate over a lifetime.
• Research Need 13: Clarify how biopsychosocial factors affect health outcomes over time in racial and ethnic groups of middle-aged and older adults.
• Research Need 14: Identify differences in health care—access, use, and quality—for racial and ethnic minority populations other than blacks.
• Research Need 15: Determine the reasons for differences in health care quality, focusing on the contributions of geographic variation, characteristics of health care institutions, provider behavior and stereotyping, and patient adherence to recommendations for care.
• Research Need 16: Place particular emphasis on panel studies that follow cohorts in order to study differences in health among racial and ethnic groups over the life course.
• Research Need 17: Measure the use of complementary and alternative therapies by racial and ethnic groups.
• Research Need 18: Characterize long-term trends (and possible lags) in the effects of changing social policy—federal, state, and local—on health differences and on public health.

1

The Nature of
Racial and Ethnic Differences

Poor health comes eventually for most people in late life. But does it start earlier, last longer, and appear more common for some racial and ethnic groups than for others? If so, what are the causes of those differences and what can interventions do to affect them? This report examines these questions.

Racial and ethnic differences in late-life health may impose societal costs, and they rub against the American grain. They suggest possible inequity in life histories and opportunities, perhaps from exposure to unhealthy environments (e.g., Faber and Krieg, 2002), or in access to or the adequacy of medical care (Institute of Medicine, 2002).

Not all health differences necessarily involve inequity, however. Some may be due to life-styles freely chosen, especially in younger years, or to attitudes toward treatment. It is important therefore to understand the roots and mechanisms of health differences and to consider ways to reverse them, or at least to alleviate further damage, with the objective of providing all individuals the opportunity for the fullest possible exercise of their capacities in late life.

In 1994 the Committee on Population of the National Research Council held a workshop on health differences in late life. The papers from that workshop, published in 1997 in a volume entitled *Racial and Ethnic Differences in the Health of Older Americans* (National Research Council, 1997), summarized existing data on racial and ethnic differences in mortality, morbidity, disability, and dementia and discussed the role of such factors as socioeconomic status, health behaviors, the social environment, the use of medical care, and genes.

Recognizing the need for continuing research, as well as the increasing diversity of the U.S. population, the National Institute on Aging (which sponsored the 1994 workshop) commissioned a new panel to update the work and develop research recommendations. The panel's specific mandate was to:

- organize a 2-day workshop with leading researchers from a variety of disciplines and professional orientations to answer questions about the nature and extent of racial and ethnic differences in health in old age, the social and biological mechanisms involved, what studies would advance understanding of differences, and what opportunities exist for research on special populations or research in special areas such as the biology and genetics of aging; and
- provide a short report summarizing the main lessons learned and providing recommendations for further work.

The panel's summary of research findings, disciplinary issues, and possibilities for future research is covered in this volume. The commissioned papers, which were presented at the panel's workshop in Washington, DC in 2002, appear in a companion volume (National Research Council, 2004; see the table of contents in the Appendix).

In addressing its charge, the panel was forced to confront a large and burgeoning theoretical and empirical literature that involves researchers from virtually all the medical, social, and behavioral sciences. The panel's initial intention was to produce a short report of the state of knowledge, but it rapidly became apparent that current research provides no simple answers. What is currently known about the origins of racial and ethnic differences in health points in many different directions. This fundamental finding spurred the panel to produce a more comprehensive and complex report than was originally requested, detailing what is currently known about apparent health differences and the role and operation of each of the major risk factors involved. This work was seen as an important prerequisite for identifying the kind of research that might advance this field.

This report and the companion volume of papers update work reported on in the papers from an earlier Committee on Population Workshop (National Research Council, 1997). Many of the issues discussed in this volume are similar to those raised in the earlier one, but seen through different lenses and with different emphases.

In this chapter we consider why we focus on racial and ethnic groups and what groups we distinguish. We then characterize the health differences in late life that have been reported among racial and ethnic groups.

These differences reveal a complicated picture that requires careful scrutiny. Chapters 2 through 11 explore the possible causes of health differences, including the social, environmental, psychological, and biological factors that may be at the root of racial and ethnic advantage or disadvantage in health. Chapter 12 asks whether and how action can deal with health differences and what the effects might be.

We refer throughout this report to differences rather than disparities, because the latter term has recently acquired a connotation of injustice, which is not always appropriate for the differences we consider, notably but not only when a minority population is actually in better health than the majority population. Although our focus is on late life, we offer some information on group differences more broadly, as context and in the absence of data on late life.

RACIAL AND ETHNIC GROUPS

Definitions

Race is a potent social reality and an important and enduring component of personal identity. In censuses and most surveys, a designation of race is selected by individual respondents from officially specified categories. This self-identification does not mean that race is without objective basis, since it is roughly consistent with ancestral origins. Yet because of the complications of migration histories and intermarriage, as well as the vagaries of self-identification and social categorization, racial classifications diverge from strict classification by descent.

Ethnicity is similar in concept to race. But while races have often been distinguished on the basis of physical characteristics, especially skin color, ethnic distinctions generally focus on such cultural characteristics as language, history, religion, and customs (Montague, 1942). However, physical and cultural characteristics are often conflated in the identification of racial and ethnic groups. What begins as an ethnic or cultural distinction often becomes racialized, and racial groups are often identified, in the public mind, with reference to customs and behavior. We generally refer here to racial and ethnic groups, without making any sharp distinction between these terms.

Five races are currently distinguished in official U.S. government statistics (Office of Management and Budget, 1997): white, black or African American, American Indian or Alaska Native, Asian, and Native Hawaiian or other Pacific Islander. An additional distinction is made between Hispanics or Latinos and all others, this being designated as an "ethnic" distinction that crosscuts the racial classification. The 2000 census followed this classification—but also allowed multiple choices—and individuals selected their own identification as they had since the 1970 census. (Such self-identification has been used in censuses since 1970, though with different categories; before that, interviewers classified respondents.)

Self-identification sometimes gives people options, depending on the context. Racial and ethnic identities vary as a function of social and psychological factors that may alter their salience (Yancey et al., 1976). For instance, with the decline of stigma and greater emphasis on the rights of indigenous peoples, the number of people who say they are American Indians or Alaska Natives has increased over time far faster than would be possible from natural increase (Harris and Sim, 2002). A questionnaire provides sample categories that also can affect individuals' choices. English was the largest ethnic group in the 1980 U.S. census, but the size of this group declined by 34 percent when it was not listed as an example in 1990 (Waters, 2000: 1730).

As self-identification has become the norm, pressure has grown to allow multiple and interracial identification, which was done in the 2000 census. When asked to choose one race, more than 80 percent of multiracial individuals will do so (Sondik et al., 2000), but given the option of multiple identities, some people choose more than one, with more educated people being more likely to do so (Lieberson and Waters, 1993). Again, this depends on context. For instance, adolescents choose multiracial identities on surveys more often at school than at home (Harris and Sim, 2002). In the 2000 census, 2.4 percent of the population chose more than one race (U.S. Census Bureau, 2002b).

The categories used by the U.S. Office of Management and Budget (OMB) are a small part of the possible racial and ethnic distinctions that might be made among Americans. An encyclopedia of immigrant groups (Levinson and Ember, 1997) provides profiles of 161 groups, from Acadians to Zoroastrians, and this does not include native groups, such as the more than 550 American Indian tribal groups recognized by the Bureau of Indian Affairs. There are of course almost an infinite number of physical and cultural characteristics that could be used to define racial and ethnic groups, and the major groups are defined with reference to a very small subset of these.

In this report we generally follow the OMB classification, with minor modifications (at least partly to accommodate earlier data and studies). We treat Hispanics as a distinct group and all other groups referred to in this report explicitly exclude Hispanics. We do not distinguish Native Hawaiians and Pacific Islanders, treating them together with Asians when the data require this or leaving them out. We treat American Indians and Alaska Natives as a single group. We do not identify Alaska Natives separately since they account for only 0.03 percent of the combined group and are not distinguished (and are probably not represented) in any of the studies we

TABLE 1-1 Population Aged 65 and Older, 2000 and Projected 2050

Racial or Ethnic Group	Number (millions)		Percent		Annual Growth Rate (%)
	2000	2050	2000	2050	2000-2050
All groups	34.84	82.00	100.0	100.0	1.71
White	29.10	52.68	83.5	64.2	1.19
Black	2.83	10.00	8.1	12.2	2.53
Hispanic	1.94	13.42	5.6	16.4	3.87
Asian or Pacific Islander	0.82	5.37	2.4	6.5	3.75
American Indian or Alaska Native	0.15	0.53	0.4	0.6	2.50

SOURCE: Estimated from U.S. Census Bureau (2002a).

covered. The five racial and ethnic groups we consider, therefore, are Hispanics, whites, blacks, Asians, and American Indians and Alaska Natives. Because of the paucity of data, we do not consider multiracial groups.

Table 1-1 shows the numbers of individuals aged 65 years or older in each of the major groups. In 2000, whites were 83.5 percent of this age group, a substantially larger proportion than their 71.4 percent in the general population. Part of the reason for the difference is the number of younger immigrants, mostly nonwhite, which reduces the proportion of whites at younger ages. The foreign-born population in the United States has become increasingly younger since the 1960s (He, 2002). Nevertheless, in the older population, the foreign born were a substantial, if not dominant, proportion in some groups in 2000. Fully 50 percent of Hispanics 65 years and older were foreign born, as well as 84 percent of Asians and Pacific Islanders (U.S. Census Bureau, 2001).

By 2050, whites are projected to be only 64.2 percent of those aged 65 and older. The Hispanic proportion will almost triple in this period, going from 5.6 to 16.4 percent, and Asians will increase almost as fast. Blacks and American Indians and Alaska Natives will show more moderate growth, but still faster growth than whites because of differential fertility in the past, delayed improvements in mortality, and population momentum (U.S. Census Bureau, 2002a). Whether these racial and ethnic distinctions will remain socially relevant cannot be predicted, but some of them have persisted for centuries. In any case, any differences in health in later life among these groups will become increasingly consequential.

Disparate Treatment

Historically, the recognition of new racial and ethnic groups in the U.S. population has often been marked by conflict, prejudice, and disparate treatment, providing a special reason for concern about the health of racial and ethnic minorities.

An early and enduring racial and ethnic distinction developed between the native American Indian inhabitants of the continent and the European colonists. Although the natives divided themselves into numerous racial and ethnic or tribal groups, for many purposes the colonists and their governments used a dichotomous distinction between themselves and the natives—a lumping together of the American Indian and Alaska Native populations that is still used in government statistics.

The forcible importation into the American colonies of Africans as slaves gave rise to a third enduring racial or ethnic category. The definition of this category has varied over time (as it does in other countries, such as Brazil and South Africa). The United States held for several centuries to a rule of hypodescent, so that any African or African American ancestry defined a person as black. For three centuries, this limited their rights under law and in practice and marked them as members of a subordinate group (Massey and Denton, 1993).

Other waves of immigration have created and continue to create separately identified racial and ethnic groups in the United States. The large European immigrations of the late nineteenth and early twentieth centuries, first from Northern and then Southern and Eastern Europe, created major new groups. At the height of this immigration, European ethnic groups were often treated as distinct races in the census and other government statistics and heavily discriminated against. For instance, the Irish were racialized first by the British (Allen, 1994) and later also in American society (Ignatiev, 1995). Racial and ethnic distinctions among Americans of European origin are now generally muted, and individuals manifest considerable variation in how much they identify with their European ancestry. This muting of distinctions is also observed in other racial and ethnic groups, though black Americans have had much less latitude than other groups.

Hispanic and Asian immigration began early, some Hispanic settlement in fact predating the accession of particular territories to the United States. Immigration has greatly accelerated in recent decades, rising to levels that rival those of the earlier massive European immigrations. Somewhat in contrast to the practices of those earlier periods, society and government, including statistical agencies and researchers, have not distinguished among the many different national origins of the Hispanic and Asian populations, which has created a set of issues and dilemmas for research. As in other waves of immigration, many Hispanics and early Asian immigrants have at least initially borne the burden of low-wage work and social inferiority (though often earning more than in their countries of origin).

Immigrant groups have immediately become part of the system of social stratification in U.S. society, generally starting at the bottom of the social ladder. Access to valued resources—jobs, income and wealth, education, power and prestige—generally comes over decades or generations. Ethnic stratification has often given rise to racist ideologies that ascribe inherent inferiority to particular groups (Van den Berghe, 1964).

How Group Membership May Affect Health

Belonging to a particular ethnic group can be linked to health in a variety of ways. Differences in genetic characteristics could produce differences in susceptibility to disease. Since racial and ethnic identity is a crucial part of personal identity, it may be associated with ways of behaving and reacting to the social environment that have implications for health. Since groups differ in their social standing—which tends to evolve over time—their access to health resources may vary. Since groups are not always treated similarly, some may experience more favorable environments for health than others. Arguably, some of these effects could be particularly notable among older people, whose racial and ethnic identification may be more deeply rooted and whose life experiences may reflect early, perhaps turbulent, history of race and ethnic relations. We consider all of these possible effects of racial and ethnic identity systematically in subsequent chapters.

Three complications in the way racial and ethnic groups are defined are important to note for their possible effects on health differences. First, self-identification allows certain biases to enter group comparisons. For instance, consider the case of American Indians and Alaska Natives. As noted earlier, their numbers have increased rapidly, at least partly because some people are identifying with this group who had not previously done so (Sandefur et al., 2004). These individuals often do not live on designated federal reservations and have higher socioeconomic status than those who do. Though such changes in self-identification need not affect individual health, they still affect average group health, in this case reducing any health disadvantage of American Indians and Alaska Natives relative to other groups. Such selection effects are considered further below.

Second, for one important health outcome—mortality—self-identification is not the norm. Funeral home directors, sometimes with information from relatives, may make the determination of race and ethnicity of the deceased. The complication, from this and other possible sources of misclassification, amounts to published death rates that are too high for whites and blacks (by 1 percent and 5 percent respectively) and too low for American Indians (21 percent), Asian and Pacific Islanders (11 percent), and Hispanics (2 percent) (Rosenberg et al., 1999). A recent study of state hospital discharge data in California found that approximately 70 percent of hospitalizations of Indian Health Service (IHS) enrolled patients were incorrectly classified as non-American Indian (Korenbrot et al., 2003; see also Grossman, 2003).

A third complication involves the way the major groups are defined. Though they reflect major social distinctions, they may or may not reflect the distinctions that are most relevant in assessing health. It is difficult to tell a priori what racial and ethnic distinctions would be most productive for health research, and some possible distinctions may involve groups too small to be studied nationally. It is important to keep in mind, however, that each of these five major groups we consider is in fact an amalgam of many smaller groups that, in a previous era, might have been separately distinguished, and that may still consider themselves distinct.

Finally, note that the relationship between group membership and health is somewhat different with regard to American Indians and Alaska Natives because of the existence of the IHS. Tribes employ very explicit eligibility criteria to define membership, which are formally ratified by the Bureau of Indian Affairs, U.S. Department of the Interior. These criteria vary among tribes, as it is within their purview to define membership, ranging from different degrees of blood quantum to other, nonconsanguineal forms of descent reckoning. Tribal enrollment, in turn, determines eligibility for access to federally sponsored health care provided through the IHS. There is a strong, but not isomorphic, relationship between tribal enrollment and residence: most American Indians/Alaska Natives living on or near reservations are enrolled tribal members, but as much as 60 percent of the enrolled population lives off-reservation, in rural, suburban, and urban areas. Relatively few individuals who self-identify as American Indian and Alaska Native but are nonenrolled in tribal registers reside in reservations. Thus, in this subpopulation, the issue of identification is not simply a psychological phenomenon but one that has enormous implications for access to health care.

DIFFERENCES IN MORTALITY AND HEALTH IN LATE LIFE

The health differences in late life among the five major groups—Hispanics, whites, blacks, Asians, and American Indians and Alaska Natives—are complex but can be briefly summarized. Blacks generally have worse health than other groups. American Indians and Alaska Natives, especially those on reservations, are also less healthy than other groups except blacks. Whites are usually taken as the standard against which other groups are compared, but they are not necessarily in the best health. Hispanics appear to be healthier than whites on a number of measures, though not all. Asians are generally in better health than any other group (Hummer et al., 2004).

These generalizations are based on various indicators of health, especially mortality rates, self-rated overall health, the prevalence of major diseases, and measures of physical and cognitive functioning (Hummer et al., 2004; Manly and Mayeux, 2004). There are consistencies across indicators; however, health is multidimensional, and the pattern of racial and ethnic differences is not uniform.

Mortality

The black disadvantage in mortality is clear. As shown in Figures 1-1 and 1-2, the official death rates for black males and females are 30-50 percent higher than those of whites at ages 65-79. Official statistics have various limitations—underregistration of deaths, disparities in racial and ethnic identification between registered deaths and the base census population, and inaccurate age reporting. However, attempts to correct for such data limitations still leave a significant black-white gap (Hummer et al., 2004). Overall, life expectancy for blacks is nearly 7 years shorter than for whites (Rogers et al., 2000), given that mortality is also higher for blacks at younger ages: more than twice that of whites among infants and still twice that of whites at ages 20-24.

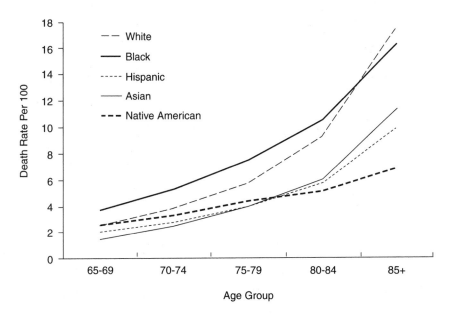

FIGURE 1-1 Death rates per 100,000 by race and ethnicity: Males 65 years and older, 1999.
SOURCE: Derived by Hummer et al. (2004) from Hoyert et al. (2001).

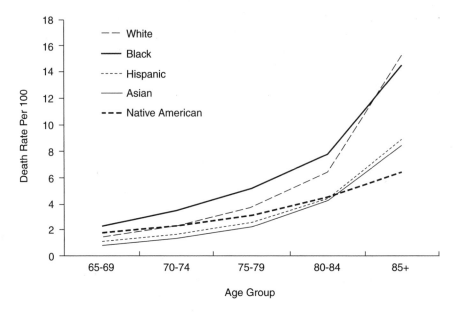

FIGURE 1-2 Death rates per 100,000 by race and ethnicity: Females 65 years and older, 1999.
SOURCE: Derived by Hummer et al. (2004) from Hoyert et al. (2001).

For other minorities, official statistics suggest that individuals 65 years and older have lower mortality rates than whites. In some cases, this minority advantage stands up under scrutiny; in others, it does not, or may still be questionable, as data limitations have been less studied among other minorities than among blacks.

Mortality rates for Hispanics appear to be biased downward, but corrected rates are still lower than those for whites. The Hispanic mortality advantage is not consistent over the life course. Hispanics have similar mortality levels to whites in infancy but 24 percent higher levels at 20-24, with this disadvantage decreasing and turning into an advantage in late adulthood (Hummer et al., 2004; Liao et al., 1998, Rogers et al., 2000). Among Hispanic subgroups, Puerto Ricans show this pattern most clearly, with a substantial mortality disadvantage relative to whites, greater than that for blacks, at ages 18-44 (whether or not socioeconomic factors are controlled), still some disadvantage at ages 45-64, and a small nonsignificant advantage at ages 65 and older (Rogers et al., 2000).

One factor to keep in mind, therefore, is the fact that comparisons at older ages only involve those who survive to these ages; thus, if mortality is higher at younger ages for Hispanics, those who survive to older ages would be a select group in some sense (we discuss this argument, which could apply to all groups, in subsequent chapters). Another factor of note is the large proportion of foreign born among Hispanics (and island born among Puerto Ricans), a proportion that varies by age and reaches its peak around age 40.

As for Hispanics, the mortality rates for Asians are biased downward, but corrected rates are still better than those for whites. In contrast to Hispanics, the Asian mortality advantage appears consistently at all ages. Notably, the proportion foreign born is even higher, at all ages, among Asians than Hispanics.

For American Indians and Alaska Natives, the apparent overall advantage over whites in mortality in old age may be entirely illusory, since their rates are estimated to be 21 percent too low (Rosenberg et al., 1999), mainly because decedents are misclassified and are particularly unreliable at the oldest ages. Somewhat more reliable data come from the IHS (1999), which covers the 60 percent of American Indians and Alaska Natives living on federal reservations or in counties near them. These data show mortality levels for those 65 years and older that are 40 percent higher than those for whites. Survey data linked to subsequent mortality information, in contrast to official death rates, also suggest that American Indian and Alaska Native mortality levels are at least similar to those for whites. Notably, American Indian and Alaska Native mortality at younger ages is substantially higher than among whites: 60 percent higher among infants and almost twice as high for those 20-24 years old (Hummer et al., 2004).

At the oldest ages, for those 85 years and older, mortality rates appear to cross over in some cases, with black mortality falling below that of whites and American Indian and Alaska Native mortality falling below that of Hispanics and Asians and Pacific Islanders (see Figures 1-1 and 1-2). The black-white crossover appears in many data sets, though skepticism persists about data quality because of such problems as age misreporting. Recent evidence still suggests a crossover at ages 90-94 for males and 95 and older for females (Hill et al., 2000). However, the crossovers involving American Indians and Alaska Natives are suspect because of data problems. A crossover also appears, as noted above, for Hispanics relative to whites, but below age 65 and therefore not shown in Figures 1-1 and 1-2.

An important factor in any actual crossover is the possibility of selection: higher mortality earlier in life could leave fewer but more robust members in some racial and ethnic groups. This could, in fact, affect comparisons for older adults as a whole, since survival to age 65 is less common among blacks and American Indians and Alaska Natives.

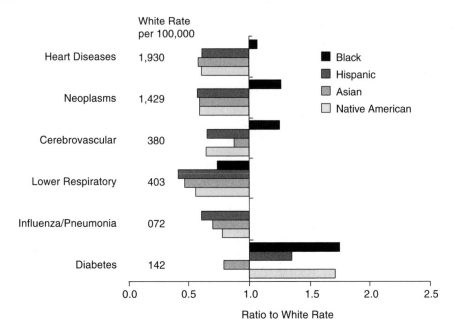

FIGURE 1-3 Death rates of racial and ethnic groups by underlying cause: Males 65 years and older, 1999.
SOURCE: Based on Anderson (2001).

Causes of Death

Figures 1-3 and 1-4 show six leading causes of death for males and females by racial and ethnic group. The rates and ratios shown are subject to the same qualifications as overall mortality rates, as well as not being age-standardized. Diseases of the heart and neoplasms are the leading underlying causes of death for every racial and ethnic group, between them accounting for over half of all deaths at age 65 and older. For other causes, rankings vary slightly by group (so that diabetes, the sixth cause shown, actually ranks lower for some groups than Alzheimer's disease).

Older blacks have higher death rates than older whites from the two leading causes, heart diseases and neoplasms. For the third cause, cerebrovascular diseases, the death rates are sharply higher among men and somewhat marginally higher among women. Blacks do die less often from the fourth and fifth causes shown—lower respiratory infections and influenza and pneumonia. But older blacks are also more likely than whites to die from diabetes, nephritis, and septicemia (Hummer et al., 2004). Data on causes of death therefore generally substantiate higher mortality among older blacks than whites.

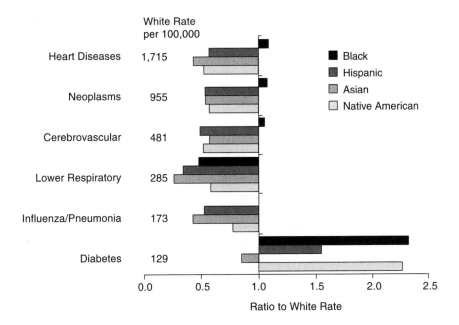

FIGURE 1-4 Death rates of racial and ethnic groups by underlying cause: Females 65 years and older, 1999.
SOURCE: Based on Anderson (2001).

In contrast to blacks, other minorities appear to be at lower risk than whites from any of the five leading causes. Only for the sixth leading cause—diabetes—do whites enjoy an advantage over Hispanics, American Indians, and Alaska Natives. Except for diabetes, the Hispanic advantage is quite general (Markides et al., 1997; Rosenwaike, 1987; Sorlie et al., 1993) and extends to the other major causes of death and even to a residual category after the ten leading causes are accounted for.

The American Indian and Alaska Native advantage appears almost as consistent (except for diabetes, as noted, and nephritis among women and accidents among men), but is not as large, and it rests on weaker data. American Indians and Alaska Natives on reservations, however, have higher cause-specific death rates than American Indians and Alaska Natives more generally, and they are also at a disadvantage relative to whites for influenza and pneumonia. The death rate on reservations at age 65 and older from influenza and pneumonia is two-and-a-half times that for American Indians and Alaska Natives generally and twice that for whites (Indian Health Service, 1999).

Lastly, Asians have lower cause-specific death rates than whites for all the leading causes, including diabetes (Hummer et al., 2004; Williams, 2001b). However, this is not the case for Pacific Islanders specifically.

Among the leading causes not shown in the figures, there is one further interesting contrast: whites have a substantially higher death rate from Alzheimer's disease than any other group. For older white women, for instance, the rate is 75 percent higher than the rate for blacks and more than double the rate for any other group (Hummer et al., 2004).

One way to summarize these contrasts, at least between whites and black, is to estimate how much each cause of death contributes to the racial and ethnic differences. We cannot look specifically at older people, but analysis has been done for all ages combined. Across all ages, deaths from hypertension contribute the most to black-white differences (15 percent), followed by HIV (11 percent), diabetes (8 percent), and homicide (8 percent) (Wong et al., 2002). At older ages, two of these causes—HIV and homicide—should be less significant, which may have some influence on the convergence of black and white mortality rates.

Health and Disability

In some respects, comparisons of health and disability across racial and ethnic groups are consistent with the mortality comparisons, but in others they are not. Surveys often ask people to rate their health as excellent, very good, good, fair, or poor, and these ratings generally correlate with subsequent mortality. Table 1-2 shows the percentages of people who report fair or poor health in pooled National Health Interview Surveys from 1989 to 1994 (Hummer et al., 2004). Though there is some variation at the oldest ages, self-rated health for blacks is generally the worst among all racial and ethnic groups (Hayward and Heron, 1999), and self-rated health for Asians is generally the best. Between these extremes, rankings are different from those for mortality. Whites have better self-rated health than Hispanics and much better self-rated health than American Indians and Alaska Natives.

Comparisons of groups in regard to activity limitations (Table 1-2) parallel those for self-rated health. The limitations indicator includes individuals who report being unable to perform their major activity, being limited in it, or being limited in other activities. The rankings by racial and ethnic groups on this indicator are essentially the same as for self-rated health, except that American Indians and Alaska Natives are worse than blacks for some age and gender categories.

In contrast to mortality rates, black and white morbidity indicators do not cross over at the oldest ages. Even at the oldest ages, blacks report more severe problems with disability and functioning than whites.

Health and disability comparisons could differ from mortality comparisons for substantive reasons, or the differences could be artifactual. The

TABLE 1-2 Self-Rated Health and Activity Limitations, Pooled 1989-1994 Data

Racial or Ethnic Group	Male			Female		
	65-74	75-84	85+	65-74	75-84	85+
Self-Rated Health: Percent Fair or Poor						
White	24.5	30.8	32.0	23.0	29.1	34.0
Black	41.3	47.3	51.4	41.0	45.8	46.2
Hispanic	—[a]	—[a]	—[a]	—[a]	—[a]	—[a]
Mexican	34.1	45.3	56.6	36.0	44.7	48.1
Other	30.0	34.6	40.3	32.0	41.7	44.9
Asian or Pacific Islander	18.2	17.4	—[a]	20.9	35.0	—[a]
American Indian and Alaska Native	35.4	51.0	—[a]	34.2	40.5	—[a]
Percent with Activity Limitations						
White	35.0	39.5	49.6	32.8	41.0	60.8
Black	41.6	48.1	59.5	43.2	51.1	65.7
Hispanic	—[a]	—[a]	—[a]	—[a]	—[a]	—[a]
Mexican	39.3	38.4	70.8	39.9	41.4	57.2
Other	36.3	35.2	51.6	34.3	47.3	68.6
Asian or Pacific Islander	22.1	32.2	30.8	20.0	33.5	43.5
American Indian and Alaska Native	44.6	36.4	—[a]	42.9	66.5	63.2

[a]Too few cases.
SOURCE: Hummer et al. (2004).

data come from different sources, and for the oldest groups they are fairly scanty. Self-reported health and disability estimates come from survey data—rather than being based on registration and census data—which exclude the institutionalized population and may miss 2-5 percent of decedents (Hummer et al., 2004). Some research suggests that, for cultural reasons, Hispanic immigrants may be more likely than others to report ill health, and their reports may be less predictive of subsequent mortality (Finch et al., 2002).

Diseases and Conditions

Reports of specific diseases and health conditions are more difficult to compare systematically across all groups than general health and disability. Some comparisons can be made, though the picture gets increasingly clouded. The 1998 National Health Interview Survey compares three groups—whites, blacks, and Hispanics—on selected diseases and conditions (Pleis and Coles, 2002). Table 1-3 shows the percentage of people aged 65 years and older in each group who report ever having been diagnosed with each condition.

Older blacks report a diagnosis of hypertension much more often than whites. This is true for both sexes, though such diagnoses are reported more

TABLE 1-3 People 65 Years and Older with a Particular Disease or Condition

Selected Diseases and Conditions	Males				Females			
	Total	Whites	Blacks	His-panics	Total	Whites	Blacks	His-panics
Circulatory Diseases								
Heart disease, total	35.9	37.6	27.9	22.9	29.2	29.9	29.0	20.4
Coronary heart disease	26.4	27.9	19.3	17.9	17.6	18.0	17.6	14.2
Hypertension	41.6	41.0	52.7	32.6	49.6	47.7	67.6	47.9
Stroke	9.7	9.6	13.1	5.8	7.2	7.1	8.4	9.6
Respiratory Diseases								
Chronic emphysema	6.8	7.1	5.9	4.2	3.8	4.1	2.2	1.3
Asthma	6.3	6.1	7.4	6.9	8.9	8.7	10.5	8.9
Hay fever	5.8	6.1	5.1	2.5	8.1	8.1	8.5	6.6
Sinusitis	11.8	12.4	9.8	9.1	18.2	18.4	20.2	14.6
Bronchitis	4.5	4.7	3.7	3.6	7.6	8.2	4.6	5.4
Types of Cancer								
Any cancer	18.6	20.1	13.0	9.6	17.3	19.0	9.3	7.8
Breast cancer	0.2	0.3	n/a	n/a	6.5	6.9	4.7	2.3
Cervical cancer	n/a	n/a	n/a	n/a	1.0	1.1	0.8	0.7
Prostate cancer	6.4	6.7	6.4	5.1	n/a	n/a	n/a	n/a
Other Diseases and Conditions								
Diabetes	13.3	12.1	17.6	19.4	13.6	11.9	26.0	21.2
Ulcers	15.6	15.6	13.9	14.7	12.3	12.3	11.9	11.4
Kidney disease	3.4	3.3	3.8	3.3	3.2	2.9	4.6	1.7
Liver disease	1.1	1.2	0.3	2.2	1.4	1.4	2.4	0.2
Arthritic symptoms	31.8	32.1	32.4	28.3	40.8	40.7	41.9	44.5

n/a, Not applicable or no data.
NOTE: Data are for people who have been told by a doctor or other health professional that they have the disease or condition.
SOURCE: 1998 National Health Interview Survey (Pleis and Coles, 2002).

frequently by women than men. Blacks also report a previous stroke more often than whites, but black males are less likely than whites to report heart disease. This is somewhat inconsistent and it should be noted that these are self-reports, and anyone who died from these diseases (or from any other cause) is not in the comparison. Blacks report a previous diagnosis of any cancer much less often than whites, including reports of breast cancer among women. Blacks report substantially more frequent diagnoses of diabetes.

These comparisons are consistent with other data in which blacks do not report any greater heart disease morbidity than whites (Crimmins et al., 2004; Hayward et al., 2000). In these data, blacks aged 50 and older report higher levels than whites of hypertension, diabetes, stroke, kidney disease, bladder problems, lung problems, asthma, back problems, foot and leg problems, and vision and hearing problems (Hayward et al., 2000). On the last problem, however, testing of adults, as well as reported diagnoses, suggest better hearing among blacks, particularly elderly black men, than whites (Desai et al., 2001; Henselman et al., 1995; Jerger et al., 1986; Pleis and Coles, 2002).

Among blacks, dementia and Alzheimer's disease appear to be more prevalent than among whites (Manly and Mayeux, 2004), despite Alzheimer's being more often listed as a cause of death for whites. Although precise comparisons of cognitive status are clearly difficult for populations with different educational backgrounds, blacks do appear more likely to suffer from vascular dementia than whites (Manly and Mayeux, 2004). In contrast, blacks report lower levels of depression than whites.

Hispanics report being diagnosed with diabetes much more often than whites, but much less often with circulatory diseases (with the exception of stroke among women) and any cancer, including breast cancer (see Table 1-3; Pleis and Coles, 2002). Some other data suggest more self-reports of respiratory problems, infections, pneumonia, influenza, and accidents (Markides and Black, 1996), though this is on the face of it inconsistent with fewer deaths from these causes among Hispanics. Levels of cognitive impairment and affective disorders for Hispanics appear to be higher than among whites, a comparison complicated by differences in socioeconomic status as well as language (Manly and Mayeux, 2004; Myers and Hwang, 2004).

There is a little more information about Mexicans in the United States than about other Hispanics. Mexicans' life expectancies are similar to those for whites (Rogers et al., 1996; Sorlie et al., 1993); they have higher levels of disability than whites or other Hispanics (Hummer et al., 2004) and are sometimes reported to be less likely to suffer from major depression (Burnam et al., 1987).

Asians are not in the data for Table 1-3, but other data show they have lower prevalence than whites for heart disease, cancer, and cardiovascular disease (Kagawa-Singer et al., 1997; Whittemore, 1989; Ziegler et al., 1993), consistent with their lower mortality levels. The evidence on relative levels of depression for Asians is mixed: some studies show Asians' reporting higher levels of depression than whites, while others find lower levels (Kuo, 1984; Myers and Hwang, 2004).

The Asian and Pacific Islander population is a composite of many groups that vary in health as well as many other life circumstances. Little is known about Asian subgroups, but research has shown Indians, Chinese,

Filipinos, and Japanese report similar or better health status than whites (Kuo and Porter, 1998), while Native Hawaiians and Samoans appear to have worse health (Hoyert and Kung, 1997). Older U.S. residents of Chinese, Filipino, Indian, Korean, and Vietnamese heritage have lower mortality than whites. Mortality rates among these groups do not follow socioeconomic rankings. For instance, Vietnamese, who have lower average incomes than Indians, have lower mortality than Indians in every age group of 65 years and older (Lauderdale and Kestenbaum, 2002).

Besides differences in broad disease categories, racial and ethnic differences exist in specific diseases. With cancer, for instance, the data show these differences (Burdette, 1998; Manton and Stallard, 1997):

- more cases of melanoma among whites than other groups;
- high rates of ovarian cancer among whites of European ancestry;
- lower incidence of breast cancer among blacks and Hispanics than other groups;
- twice as many cases of cervical cancer among blacks than among all other groups, though not among those aged 65 years and older, and higher incidence among Hispanics than non-Hispanics (Armstrong et al., 2002);
- a high incidence of pancreatic cancer among blacks and those of Polynesian ancestry;
- lower rates of cancers of the gallbladder and cystic ducts among blacks than other groups; and
- a higher risk of multiple myeloma among blacks than whites.

Differences also exist within the major racial and ethnic groups. Among Asians, for instance, breast cancer incidence is twice as high among Japanese as among Vietnamese women; in contrast, cervical cancer incidence is seven times as high among Vietnamese as among Japanese women (Miller et al., 1996; Williams, 2001b).

Knowledge about all these differences is limited by numerous problems of measurement. For instance, the ethnicity of decedents may not be reliably determined, because it must be reported by someone else. For other health indicators, ethnic identification could be more accurate, though people may be inconsistent in reporting their own race or ethnic status, particularly when they are of mixed descent. Health status may also be reported inconsistently. For instance, disability is often defined relative to normal activities, which may vary from group to group. Groups accustomed to more physically challenging work may report greater disability than other groups. Reports of medical conditions may be affected by the amount of contact with providers of medical care. Racial and ethnic groups with more access to the medical system may report more health problems simply because of greater contact. And there are special problems in comparing mental health across racial and ethnic groups. Finally, we have mainly compared disease prevalence across groups, but groups may also differ in such other factors as age at disease onset, duration, and severity.

NEEDED RESEARCH

The uncertainties and inconsistencies in this sketch of mortality and health differences suggest various directions for future research: to clarify the health status at older ages of particular groups, to define more clearly what appear to be contradictions in particular areas of health and disease, and to resolve apparent conflicts between indicators.

Research Need 1: Attempt a systematic decomposition of racial and ethnic health differences in mortality and morbidity among older people to determine the relative contribution of particular diseases and conditions. Try to assign differences in the prevalence of specific diseases and conditions to differences in the prevalence of major risk factors.

Racial and ethnic differences in mortality have in fact been decomposed in relation to various diseases and conditions with reference to people of all ages (Wong et al., 2002). A focus on older people would be useful. Moving beyond such decomposition to assess the contribution of risk factors of all types to differences would be a complex exercise, though perhaps a more manageable challenge than the World Health Organization's (2002) attempt to assess the contribution of all major risk factors to the global disease burden. If such partitioning can be accomplished, it should be possible to refine the research agenda to focus on the most critical areas.

The health disadvantages of blacks and American Indians and Alaska Natives appear to be the most troubling. Black disadvantages are the best documented, so the research emphasis for blacks might be more appropriately on understanding differences, which we consider in subsequent chapters.

Research Need 2: Clarify the contrasts between mortality rankings and morbidity rankings, particularly between older whites and Hispanics, and assess the relative contributions of diseases and conditions to differences in mortality and overall health.

One problematic contrast is the consistently poorer self-reported health among Hispanics than would appear warranted by mortality levels. Another is the higher incidence of heart disease mortality among blacks than whites, despite the higher reported diagnoses of the disease among whites. To understand such apparent contradictions, it would be useful to be able to assess, on a continuing basis, how much each disease or condition adds to mortality or detracts from overall health, as has been done for the population as a whole (Wong et al., 2002) but not for older adults or different ethnic groups. Some of the differences between mortality and morbidity indicators appear to vary by age group. Although various explanations are possible, such as differences in the proportion of recent immigrants across age groups, there is as yet no adequate support for any explanation.

In sorting out the possible discrepancies in group comparisons, measurement and other methodological issues require continued attention. For instance, misclassification has an important effect on statistics for some minority groups; ethnic identification and misidentification therefore need further study. The reliability and comparability of such measures as self-reported health require continued attention. Issues such as the black-white mortality crossover at the oldest ages have received much attention from demographers attempting to sort out the methodological issues. Other examples of apparent crossover, or at least convergence, also exist, as well as cases—such as with black-white morbidity—for which rates do not converge.

For some group and subgroup comparisons, inconsistencies may not be evident simply because of the lack or weakness of data. For older American Indians and Alaska Natives, for instance, higher mortality than average may or may not be a problem: the data are too uncertain to be sure. Levels of disability and specific conditions, such as diabetes, indicate health problems in this population. American Indians and Alaska Natives living on or near reservations appear to be in poorer health than others in the group. The small size of the group, however—150,000 American Indians and Alaska Natives are aged 65 and older—makes national samples less practical, though it should be feasible to study representative samples of those living on or near reservations.

Similar attention may be needed to establish the health status of other selected subgroups. This is especially true of the Hispanic and Asian groups, which are known to be heterogeneous with respect to health. Native Hawaiians, for instance, who appear to have high levels of diabetes, need to be distinguished from other Asians, who are the least likely to die of diabetes among the major groups. Subgroups can be small and costly to study, even if the focus is regional rather than national. Rather than considering all subgroups, the focus should be on subgroups that theory and prior research suggest are in substantially poorer health than the general population. As much use as possible should be made of existing data sets.

Research Need 3: When particular diseases are especially prevalent for specific racial and ethnic groups, collect more indicators of biological and functional performance in order to identify possibilities for intervention.

One area of functioning that deserves attention is differences among groups in cognitive ability and other aspects of mental health. Research would require development of measurement approaches that take account of differences in language, culture, and education among older people. Although differences in cognitive ability often mimic those in physical disability and disease, some differences do not fit this pattern. Hispanics perform worse on cognitive tests than might be expected given their life expectancy levels. In addition, previous results in this area have often been contradictory. This is partly due to reliance on nonrepresentative samples, but may also be due to tests for cognitive impairment that are not culturally sensitive. Traditional scales for indicating depression may also need to be modified for work focusing on older persons of different racial and ethnic groups (Turvey et al., 1999). Future developments in neuropsychiatric assessment and imaging techniques may help control for the effects of education and language in cognitive assessment.

Comparisons among groups, extending beyond the five major groups, might be useful in suggesting what aspects or consequences of racial and ethnic identity are really critical for health and disease and what additional dimensions should be measured. Some comparisons might involve multiracial or multiethnic groups. Study of black-white unions, for instance, suggests that the race of the mother is more important than the race of the father for infant health (Polednak and King, 1998). Other comparisons might involve racial and ethnic groups in other societies. For instance, immigrant groups in the United States lose their health advantage over time; this does not appear to be true in the United Kingdom (Nazroo, 2004), which raises important questions about mechanisms. To take another example, deaths from respiratory conditions in South Africa are considerably less common among blacks than whites (Bradshaw et al., 2004), suggesting a parallel with the U.S. situation and the possibility of investigating possible protective factors cross-nationally.

Why racial and ethnic differences in health exist is obviously a central issue for further research. The existence of some health differences may be clear, but their meaning is not. The relatively high mortality of blacks and the relatively low mortality of Asians and Hispanics give rise to several possible lines of investigation. Research on the selection of immigrants by health status may help clarify some differences involving these groups. Socioeconomic factors obviously differentiate groups and play a role in health differences, but how much of a role, and in what ways do such factors contribute? Differences at older ages require study of cohort selectivity and the effect of differential mortality on the characteristics of survivors. We consider these and other possible roots of differences in the following chapters.

Is there any basis, from looking at differences, for deciding which health differences especially need to be explained? Various plausible arguments might be made. For instance, it is important to understand the factors limiting the health of groups that are both relatively large and in the poorest health or at greatest risk of illness relative to the general population. This would certainly include black and American Indians and Alaska Natives, but also significant portions of other racial and ethnic groups. Another priority might be explaining differences that go in unexpected directions or are of unexpected size. If, for instance, the reasons for the Asian advantage in mortality and the more limited Hispanic advantage could be understood, that might provide hints about how to improve population health generally. Such arguments need not exclude research attention to other health differences, whether for theoretical or practical reasons, and would have to be qualified by what is not known yet about health differences. We briefly consider arguments about the importance of differences before turning to explanatory factors.

WHY HEALTH DIFFERENCES MATTER

The main reasons for concern about health differences are their relationship to the well-being of individuals and to society as a whole. These two concerns are different and sometimes even at odds: in some circumstances, for instance, societal well-being might demand that individuals be quarantined, whether or not this is beneficial to their own health.

What is an individual's well-being? Beyond health and economic well-being generally, it includes many other important dimensions, such as physical security, the freedom to participate in society, love and companionship, and the sense of being treated fairly. All such dimensions of well-being should be considered together, but we concern ourselves here, for illustration, with the health and income dimensions. There are important complementarities between health and income. Health is needed to earn income, and to enjoy it. Income is needed to ensure health, and people with lower incomes suffer from worse health and live shorter lives. Health and income should not be thought of as two separate contributors to well-being; they are intimately connected. Physical functions are involved in almost all aspects of earning a living and consuming goods, and health problems have different effects on different activities.

Many people care about the well-being of individuals, and many care particularly about those who have the lowest levels of well-being (Rawls, 1971). In the United States, the income component of well-being varies by race; black earnings and incomes are lower than white earnings and incomes, for example. Health differences show the same pattern. As a result, the racial gap in either income alone or health alone understates the racial gap in well-being (Deaton, 2002). In addition, blacks in the United States have historically suffered from deprivations beyond income and health, particularly deprivations of civil rights. Given this background of historical and current deprivation in multiple dimensions, racial differences in health are less tolerable than they would be if the history were more benign, and their documentation and remediation are more important.

It is important to recognize that the same arguments may not apply with equal force to all minority groups. For example, the household incomes and health of some Asian groups exceed those of native-born non-Hispanic whites. Similarly, while Hispanic incomes are similar to those of blacks and are well below those of the white majority, Hispanic health is currently, on particular though not all indicators, at least as good as that of the white majority. On such grounds, it is appropriate to distinguish among ethnic and racial minorities when evaluating the case for reducing health differences. In particular, the argument for reducing the health disadvantages of blacks is quite compelling.

There is also a separate argument about process, primarily, but not exclusively, in the provision of health care (Deaton, 2002; Sen, 2001). The extent to which health care contributes to health status is debated, but it is reasonable to suppose that some part of the variation in individuals' health status is attributable to variations in health care. If access to or quality of health care is unfairly linked to racial or ethnic identity, it deserves a remedy. This would be true even if the role of health care in maintaining health or improving longevity could not be conclusively demonstrated. Unfairness is not eliminated because its consequences are hard to demonstrate. Racial and ethnic differences in health care could be a social problem even if there were no differences in health across racial and ethnic groups, or if, for some other reason, the group that was adversely affected had superior health outcomes. Some Americans are also denied access to jobs, or housing, or are treated disrespectfully because of their race or ethnicity. These differences are of concern in their own right, and, like unequal health care, may also affect health, although the evidence that discrimination is involved in the variation in care and produces health differences remains uncertain and controversial.

These two arguments imply that black-white health differences and American Indian and Alaska Native-white health differences may be of particular concern. This is in part because blacks and American Indians and Alaska Natives have suffered, and in some cases continue to suffer, other deprivations that make their relatively poor health. There is reason to suspect that differences in health care may contribute to their inferior health, either because areas where blacks and American Indians and Alaska Natives live are served less well, or because of medically different treatment. But individual differences in preferences and choices may also be contributing factors. The health differences of other racial or ethnic groups may also be of particular concern: examples might include American Indian and Alaska Native on reservations, Native Hawaiians, and Puerto Ricans. These arguments apply to health inequalities in general, in addition to those involving race and ethnicity. For example, there is a large literature on health differences across income, wealth, and educational groups, showing that the poor typically have far worse health than the rich. (Concern about such inequalities is often greater in other countries than in the United States [Gwatkin, 2000; Independent Inquiry into Inequalities in Health, 1998]).

It is often argued that health inequities—including those across racial and ethnic groups—are important because they identify lives that can be saved. If there is no "biological" reason why poor people should be sicker than rich people or why blacks or American Indians and Alaska Natives should be sicker than whites, Hispanics, or Asians, then Americans who are poor or black or from native populations are obvious targets for health interventions. Yet it is not clear whether such targeting is the most effective way, from a medical standpoint, of improving population health.

One issue that naturally arises when group differences in health are discussed is the question of within-group heterogeneity in health. The need for health care is best identified by health status, not by membership in a socioeconomic or racial or ethnic group. Many poor people are not sick, and many rich people are. If the objective is to improve health, one should simply select people by their need for care, not by their socioeconomic status or ethnicity. In many cases, though, selecting on health status may be too late to do much good. If the goal is to prevent a disease or health-threatening condition, one needs to select people at risk, and although race or ethnicity is never the sole relevant risk factor, it is often a major risk factor. So, for example, a strategy for reducing hypertension or diabetes may target racial or ethnic groups that are at high risk for those conditions once other risk factors have been taken into account.

It is also worth asking why health differences matter from a research perspective. For example, it costs money to collect data on health differences, especially for small, hard-to-sample ethnic groups, and policy makers must decide whether or when public support for such efforts is justified. Policy priorities also depend to some extent on what causes health differences, so that it becomes an important goal of research to uncover mechanisms. For example, some people argue that health differences that are "chosen," through differences in behaviors, are a less important issue for public policy than are differences that are involuntary or that are imposed by other people's behavior. In particular, if research shows that black-white health differences are in large part attributable to differences in health care, the policy agenda would be much clearer than it currently is. One good reason for caring about black-white health differences is the possibility that this might be the case, that there are more "preventable" deaths among minorities, and that some relatively straightforward policies could bring the health of blacks closer to that of whites. The extent to which health care differences are in fact responsible for health differences between groups is an urgent research priority.

Ethnic differences in health also generate a basic research agenda. Currently, researchers are far from agreement on the causes of health differences. A good example of such an issue is the Hispanic health paradox (the high levels of Hispanic health relative to their incomes) and the effects on health of the length of time that Hispanics remain in the United States. While these may not be first-order issues given the relatively good health of Hispanics in general, they are fundamental scientific questions concerning the social determinants of health.

These arguments have a number of implications for thinking about reducing health differences. First, it is important to see reductions of health inequalities within a context of improving health more generally. Some health innovations that are clearly a good thing might exacerbate racial health differences. Thus evaluating health policies exclusively on the basis of their impact on racial and ethnic health differences would obviously be a mistake. But to say that we care about these health differences also means that, at least along the race or ethnic dimension, we should as a society be willing to devote significant additional resources to reducing the black-white gap in health outcomes.

2

Perspectives on
Racial and Ethnic Differences

The health differences we have considered present a complex picture, with older adults in some racial and ethnic groups clearly disadvantaged, though not on every dimension, and other older adults healthier than one would expect from their socioeconomic status. These differences are rooted in a complex of interlocking factors. This chapter reviews some previous attempts to analyze the evidence on differences, attempts that lead to a comprehensive framework within which these factors can be viewed. This previous work suggests variations in disciplinary perspectives, as well as possible alternative interpretations. The next nine chapters then focus on specific factors and summarize the current state of the evidence that they contribute to racial and ethnic differences; we offer recommendations about the needed research in each area.

MAJOR FACTORS

The roots of health differences, according to the summary of a 1992 national conference on behavioral and sociocultural perspectives on ethnicity and health, lie in five broad categories of factors (Anderson, 1995):

- macrosocial influences: culture, institutions and politics, media, socioeconomic status, residence, family;
- behavioral risk factors that produce chronic disease: diet, exercise, smoking, alcohol;

- risk taking and abusive behaviors that are related to infectious disease and injury: sexual practices, injury risk behavior, violent behavior, drug abuse;
- adaptive health behaviors: coping strategies, protective cultural practices, social support; and
- health care behavior: the utilization or avoidance of health care, health care seeking behavior, self-care practices, provider behavior, the doctor-patient relationship, adherence to medical regimens.

In this list, behavioral factors receive the most attention, though institutional and social factors are not ignored.

Other perspectives provide more differentiation among the nonbehavioral factors that produce differences. Hummer et al. (1998), for instance, distinguish

- socioeconomic status: education, income, wealth, employment, and occupational status;
- other social factors: marital status, marital transitions, social participation and support, nativity, religion; and
- macrosocial environment: residential factors, household factors.

These factors are assumed to operate through sets of "proximate determinants" of disease and mortality, including behavioral, psychosocial, and biological factors and health care.

Different disciplines obviously emphasize different classes of determinants of disease. We did not seek to integrate these into a unified framework, but we do need a heuristic classification within which factors at the root of differences can be reviewed and research priorities assessed. A more complete starting point than the preceding lists is a review by Kington and Nickens (2001), who investigate racial and ethnic differences in health in the United States at all ages. They do not provide a conceptual framework, but in Figure 2-1 we represent the factors they review diagrammatically. These factors include those already noted and go beyond them. Genetic factors are added as relevant to specific disease differences. Acculturation is introduced as a factor that affects health risk behavior over time. Racism and discrimination are included among psychosocial factors, particularly as possible sources of stress. Stress is one of two broad physiological conditions—the other being obesity—that are discussed and can be assumed to partly mediate the effects of behavior and psychosocial factors on health. Kington and Nickens (2001) also note the possibility that disease and disability may itself affect socioeconomic status.

The rest of this section outlines the nine factors that are covered in Chapters 3-11. The second section of this chapter briefly discusses the issue

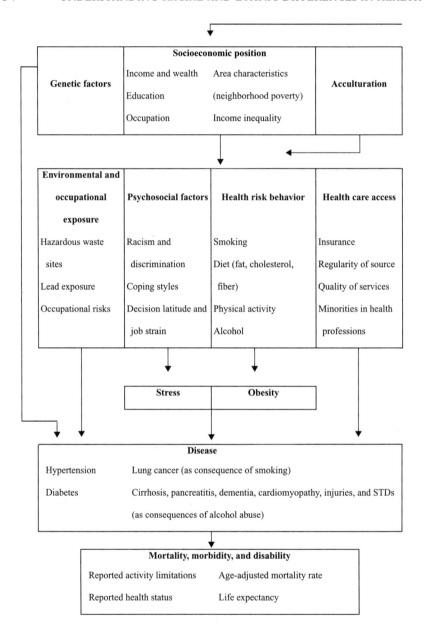

FIGURE 2-1 Factors in racial and ethnic differences in adult health.
NOTES: Most factors have a longitudinal dimension, affecting (and sometimes being affected by) health over the life course. Genetic effects on smoking are also noted by Kington and Nickens but are not represented.
SOURCE: Based on the discussion of Kington and Nickens (2001: 253-310).

of evidence for the factors. The final section considers the critical and often overlooked issue of selection, which affects all studies and analyses of differences in health in late life.

Genetic predispositions underlie the mechanisms involved in health and disease, but whether these vary sufficiently by racial and ethnic groups is a question considerably complicated by multiple factors, such as the fact that racial and ethnic groups are not strict genetic groupings and the dependence of gene action on environmental factors. While some genetic variability across races and ethnic groups is tied to vulnerability to particular diseases (e.g., Neel, 1997), the variability within groups is considerable. Single-gene disorders make a trivial contribution to overall health differences (Cooper and David, 1986). Nevertheless, gene-gene and gene-environment interactions could play an important role in differences in specific diseases.

Among other factors, it is clear that socioeconomic status is implicated in racial and ethnic health differences. We have noted multiple dimensions of status recognized in the literature, chief among them education and income and wealth. The complications in the effects of status involve not only its reciprocal relationship with health, but also nonlinearities in its effects. For older persons, socioeconomic status over their lifetimes may be relevant for current health.

One possible route of influence of socioeconomic status is through health risk behavior, which covers such important factors as diet, smoking, exercise, sexual risk taking, and drug abuse. These behaviors may have an impact on health at specific stages in the life course, such as in adolescence, or may have a cumulative effect, in either case extending their influence into later life and affecting differences at older ages.

Possibly offsetting health risk behaviors may be positive factors: personal resources and social support may provide various ways of coping with unfavorable circumstances, such as avoiding physical or mental illness or mitigating its severity. For instance, religious involvement or a sense of personal control may contribute to psychological resilience and help avoid depression. To take another example, support from relatives or other caregivers is helpful in illness or disability, although the effects on differences are not necessarily straightforward.

While other people may contribute to an individual's health through providing social support, they may also contribute to disease through prejudice and discriminatory behavior. Such behavior may also be characterized as racism, though we assume that it could be triggered not only by race but also by immigrant status, nativity, or religion. The roles of prejudice and discrimination may be broader than represented in Figure 2-1, since they can also affect such other factors as socioeconomic status, neighborhood conditions, and access to appropriate health care (e.g., Byrd and Clayton, 2002; Williams, 2001b). Researchers have focused more recently on the possibility that experiences of prejudice and discrimination may have direct effects on health, which requires specific attention.

Stress is an important consequence of the experience of prejudice and discrimination. As suggested by Figure 2-1, stress can be treated as a separate factor, potentially mediating the effects on health not only of prejudice and discrimination, but also of other social and behavioral factors. It may, for instance, result from low socioeconomic status, and it may be alleviated by personal coping skills.

Figure 2-1 does not suggest any specific mechanisms to integrate the influences of all of these preceding factors on health. Relatively recently, various biopsychosocial mechanisms have been suggested that link environmental pressures, stress, psychological reactions, and physiological responses. While the investigation of these mechanisms has not so far focused strongly on racial and ethnic variation, the potential for insight into such differences merits separate discussion of this factor.

Health care is the final factor to consider. Several dimensions of care, as suggested above, might be relevant for differences: not only access to care, but also its quality; not only the behavior of health care providers, but also patient adherence to medical regimens; not only health care seeking behavior, but also self-care practices. While socioeconomic factors may be important in variations in health care use, other cultural factors specific to racial and ethnic groups, as well as geographic and other variation in health care, may also be involved.

All of these factors may operate at different points in the life course and also have direct effects on health in late life. The life-course perspective is discussed in the final chapter on factors. It is important for understanding late-life differences, many of which may have their origin in experiences early in life, perhaps in childhood or even infancy. A life-course perspective does not identify additional factors responsible for differences beyond those already noted, but it focuses on their operation at different stages in life and on the long-term effects. In discussing all the factors, therefore, we do not focus narrowly on their operation in late life but more broadly on their operation over the life course, with implications for late-life differences.

NATURE OF THE EVIDENCE

As the study of racial and ethnic differences in health has moved away from descriptive studies towards trying to identify the underlying determinants of these differences, researchers have naturally become increasingly interested in developing models of causal processes.

Establishing causality in the social sciences is very difficult at best and in some cases impossible. A basic constraint is that the effect of anything (but say, for example, a series of stressful events) on health cannot be established without invoking some minimum assumptions or restrictions. This is because of the impossibility of observing the counterfactual (i.e., observing that individual if he or she had not been subject to that particular series of stressful events). Yet if we want to understand the impact of various policies or say anything meaningful about the relative importance of various determinants, we need to be able to make statements about plausible causality.

Even the best social science has important limitations. Good natural experiments are few and far between and it is difficult if not impossible to control for all relevant aspects of context simultaneously. Furthermore, much of the empirical literature apparently relevant to understanding the determinants of racial and ethnic differences in health is not based on solid experimental data but rather it is based on associations among observable qualitative and quantitative data.

Conversations on causality both within and across disciplines are not always easy (Bachrach and McNicoll, 2003; Moffitt, 2003). There is no settled and accepted set of principles for addressing causal questions within the social sciences and different disciplines have different levels of tolerance for various kinds of assumptions. Plausible causality is best established by combining clear models of behavior with high-quality data. Findings that have been replicated in a number of studies using a multiplicity of different approaches are usually the most convincing.

The evidence we consider on these factors comes from studies of different types—each with their own sets of strengths and weaknesses—reflecting not only the variety of disciplines interested in the nexus between health, aging, and race and ethnicity, but also the wide assortment of research questions that must be considered. To verify differences between groups, either reliable vital registration (for mortality) or large representative surveys are needed. To explain these differences, one approach that researchers take, understandably, is to investigate variables in the same large surveys. This has the presumed advantage that accurately measured differences are being explained, but it also has a number of disadvantages. The variables available may not include all those of interest, or their measures may not be the most appropriate. Racial and ethnic identification may be problematic. The racial and ethnic groups of interest, if they are minorities and have not been properly oversampled, may be represented by too few cases.

These disadvantages might be overcome with a survey specifically designed to investigate differences, but other disadvantages are inherent in studies that rely on analysis of data from even well-planned surveys. Such studies are nonexperimental, and interpreting the empirical associations that may be uncovered is not straightforward. Causal inferences drawn from such associations are hazardous. Relationships may be spurious: a given determinant and the health outcome under analysis may appear linked because both are separately related to a third factor. This possibility is a familiar problem in survey analysis: it is often addressed by taking care to include, in a multivariate model, measures of other factors that may affect the relationship under study—such as measures of socioeconomic status because of how it varies across racial and ethnic groups. Researchers can never be certain, however, that they have included all such relevant factors.

Another problem is that the temporal ordering between a presumed determinant and the health outcome of interest may not be determinable from survey data. The possibility of reverse or reciprocal causation, as suggested in the relationship between socioeconomic status and health, cannot be excluded. This problem plagues cross-sectional surveys and can even be a problem in some longitudinal designs.

A third problem involves the universe of respondents under study. Health-related factors may modify the racial and ethnic composition of this universe, which would affect any inferences about health determinants based on samples drawn from this universe. This issue, involving what are referred to as selection processes, has already been noted and will be considered in more detail shortly.

The evidence about factors in health differences is not limited to survey work. Experimental and quasi-experimental designs are also possible for addressing some issues, though not all. Not amenable to experimental study are such questions as how much prejudice and discrimination (with their potential health effects) are experienced by different racial and ethnic groups. However, experimenters do sometimes find ways to manipulate the experience of prejudice or discrimination or create laboratory analogues to such experience (Harrell et al., 2003) in order to assess the health effects. Such experimental studies have their limitations, in a sense the obverse of those of survey studies. One may question whether any specific experimental treatment can duplicate actual experience, particularly the cumulation of experience over a lifetime, and whether the small samples typically available to experimenters can provide findings that generalize to often heterogeneous racial and ethnic groups. In addition, experimental subjects may be college students rather than older persons, making the applicability of findings to older populations uncertain.

We consider in the next nine chapters the variety of studies that have been done on each major factor, trying to take the quality of the evidence into account. We note, where it is appropriate and not obvious, where conclusions are based on nonexperimental evidence or, contrariwise, on experiments of limited scope. These are not the only methodological issues, however. Issues of ethnic identification and measurement have already been noted. We will shortly consider selection issues, which could call into question findings from either survey or experimental studies. In this short summary of a diverse literature, we cannot provide a thorough methodological critique. The reader is referred to National Research Council (2004) where some specific factors and studies are treated in more detail.

SELECTION PROCESSES

Any analysis of racial and ethnic differences in health must take into account the effects of selection processes. Groups being compared will always be selected in some sense: for instance, they will necessarily be made up only of those who survive to the time of the study. This selectivity affects comparisons of group health, and it should therefore be explicitly attended to so that health differences are properly interpreted. (Selection, in the sense we use it here, is not the same thing as Darwinian selection and does not involve the evolution of genetic endowments).

Selection processes appear under various names in the literature, sometimes being referred to as unmeasured heterogeneity or drift and sometimes being labeled with reference to specific selection factors, as in "healthy migrant bias" (Abraido-Lanza et al., 1999). Related processes known as endogeneity or reciprocal causation are basically similar. The underlying processes, which can be represented within the same framework (Palloni and Ewbank, 2004), are potentially ubiquitous and need to be dealt with explicitly in interpreting health differences.

Selection Through Accession to Social Groups

Selection processes operate for any group—racial or ethnic, socio-economic, religious, residential, or any other—if joining the group is dependent on factors that also affect health and mortality. Membership in the group may subsequently affect health, but initial selection into the group will have a separate, prior, and possibly large effect.

It is indeed possible to *join* a racial or ethnic group, by self-identification, for instance. This is perhaps most relevant for those of mixed ancestry who can choose their group. If healthier individuals self-identify with one group rather than another, that might not affect their health, but it will affect group health statistics.

A more important instance of accession to a group is immigration, through which one acquires, in effect, a new identity in a new society. The case of immigration provides a good example of a selection process, resulting in the so-called "Hispanic paradox." As noted in Chapter 1, Hispanic immigrants in the United States are generally in better health than whites despite lower socioeconomic status. This paradox may be partly explained by the fact that immigrants who succeed in entering and staying in the United States seem to be drawn disproportionately from the ranks of those with better health in their countries of origin. This phenomenon is generally known as the healthy migrant effect and appears to apply even more strongly to non-Hispanic immigrants, who immigrate at greater cost from longer distances. This positive selection is stronger for immigrants of working age; weaker for children, who generally immigrate as dependents; and possibly even reversed for the oldest immigrants, who may move specifically to obtain medical care (Jasso et al., 2004).

Selection processes could also operate through socioeconomic factors, affecting groups differently and therefore having some effect on differences. For instance, individuals who develop disabilities early in life may be precluded from certain occupations. Poor health in early life may reduce the chances for higher education and more successful careers, which in turn affect health. Individuals may self-select into higher- or lower-status occupations: black children, for instance, aspire less often than white children to higher status jobs, which they associate with whites (Bigler et al., 2003).

In addition, the choice of a place of residence (whether the choice is personally made or forced on one) could lead to a selection effect if this choice is somehow related to one's health status. Aspects of residential location or neighborhood, it is argued (Morenoff and Lynch, 2004), have consequences, represented in survey analysis by "community" or "contextual" effects on health that are additional to the effects of individual characteristics. Choice of neighborhood may therefore have implications for health and may also have some link to prior health. For instance, more successful members of a minority group (who are presumably healthier) may move into more integrated neighborhoods, which would mean that any sample based on geographical concentrations of that minority would miss these healthier members and be unrepresentative of the entire group.

Selection Through Survival

As shown in Chapter 1, the magnitude and even the direction of health and mortality differences between groups change with age. A selection effect could be at work. Assume, first, that individuals are heterogeneous with regard to at least one health-related trait. (The term used in the mortality literature for such unspecified, unmeasured traits as a group is "frailty.") Then, a racial or ethnic group subject to a harsher environment than another group will lose more of its members, generally the more frail ones, over time. Gradually, this group will come to be dominated by individuals who have superior health. By some indeterminate age, the mortality disadvantage this group suffers from may diminish, or even disappear or be reversed (Manton and Stallard, 1984; Vaupel and Yashin, 1985; Vaupel et al., 1979; Yashin et al., 1999).

Such a change in mortality differences as a cohort ages is not the result of changes in behavior or environment, but simply the outcome of the fact that, over a long enough period, only healthier individuals survive. Note that this process does not require any initial difference in health-related traits between groups or any difference in the distribution of such traits within groups. The groups could be, at the start, entirely identical in frailty; over the life course, they would have been subject to different environmental pressures.

A good example of this phenomenon is the so-called black-white mortality crossover (Manton and Stallard, 1984; see Figures 1-1 and 1-2 in Chapter 1) and similar apparent crossovers for other groups. These crossovers are not necessarily just selection effects, however. They may be partly due to data artifacts, such as a greater tendency among older blacks than whites to overstate their ages.

Besides its involvement in crossovers, selection through survival could affect other health differences, though most research has paid little attention to this. For instance, it is reported that blacks are more resistant than whites to hearing loss (Henselman et al., 1995; Jerger et al., 1986) and to immunosuppression after kidney and liver transplantation (Nagashima et al., 2001). Selection could have some role in such differences, but the possibility has not been investigated.

In a cohort studied from birth (or preferably conception) to death, one need not treat selection effects separately but could, in principle, incorporate in the analysis the appropriate traits and the environmental factors that vary across groups. However, analysis of any sample of adults—and especially a sample of older people—must deal with this as a selection problem. Thorough knowledge of and complete data on the relevant traits and environmental conditions that determine survival at younger ages would permit the analysis needed to remove the influence on group composition of selection through survival. Such knowledge and data do not now exist.

Reciprocal Causation

Reciprocal causation, unlike selection processes, operates during, rather than before, the period under study. One might in fact characterize selection processes as a type of reciprocal causation that occurs before the analyst can collect any data. Technically, both can be treated in the same framework.

An example of reciprocal causation is what is referred to as "salmon bias," the return of immigrants to their countries of origin. Return migration may be occasioned by ill health, and, to the extent it is, leaves the remaining group apparently healthier. In such a case, comparing those who remain to groups of nonmigrants is misleading. This is especially a problem in studies of Hispanics. Hispanic return migration is relatively high, at least partly because Mexicans in the United States, in particular, have easier access than other immigrants to their places of origin, and their immigrant status does not constitute a political impediment to returning. Salmon bias is the obverse of healthy migrant bias and tends to reinforce the Hispanic advantage.

Changes in health status could also affect decisions about labor supply, consumption patterns, and wealth dilution that alter social standing, giving rise to another type of reciprocal causation. For example, adults affected by a health shock may incur large out-of-pocket expenses and be unable to work. When antecedent health status affects labor force participation, occupation, or wealth in this way, comparisons of health status across groups become more challenging. This process may reinforce differences between groups, as low status in a particular group gives rise to poorer health, which in turn may limit income-generating activities. In addition, the reactions of different groups may vary. The magnitude of a shock induced by equivalent health events on individuals may differ across ethnic groups, who may be exposed to contrasting labor market experiences, dissimilar health insurance coverage, and different dynamics of wealth accumulation processes. If so, reciprocal causation may leave different imprints in the patterns of health and mortality of different racial and ethnic groups.

Some of the literature refers to reciprocal causation as "direct" selection (West, 1991). This sets up a contrast with "indirect" selection, a term this literature applies to selection through accession to social positions or through survival. These terms are confusing to use, but they do help emphasize the similarities between what we have labeled selection and reciprocal causation, the latter being different mainly by taking place during rather than prior to the stage of life under study. For instance, if one could focus only on a stage of life after all return migration had taken place, then salmon bias would constitute a selection effect rather than reciprocal causation. Similarly, the effect of health on socioeconomic status may be either a selection effect, if it takes place prior to the stage of life under study, or reciprocal causation, if it takes place during this stage.

Implications

All of these selection processes are produced by a similar mechanism in that the initial composition of a group is affected by prior health and mortality conditions. The health status of the group at any given time, therefore, should not be construed as resulting solely from factors that spring from group membership. To infer the effects of group membership, one would need to remove the contribution of prior health conditions that influence membership. In order to do this, one would have to introduce factors responsible for selection into any model for interpreting racial and ethnic differences.

These selection processes should not be considered as distorting some deeper reality. The Hispanic mortality advantage, for instance, is not an illusion and is not negated by the possibility of its being rooted in selection. Rather, to the extent the selection explanation is correct, this advantage needs to be properly interpreted. The inferences to be drawn from observing such facts may not be the obvious ones. One should not assume advantageous Hispanic cultural practices or favorable behavioral profiles. By the same argument, the convergence of black and white mortality in old age (after removing the effects of data errors) is not an artifact or mirage. But because it may be partly due to selection, it does not necessarily mean either that older blacks are taking as good care of themselves or receive as satisfactory health care as whites.

Different selection processes can occur together. For instance, health differences between immigrant groups and the native population will be affected by both migration selection and survival selection (Palloni and Morenoff, 2001; Swallen, 1997). The initial immigrant advantage in mortality could expand, before contracting at the oldest ages. An increasing short-term advantage could occur if immigrant groups rapidly lose their most frail members as a result of exposure to unfamiliar risks, while native groups experience only average losses of frail individuals.

The literature on race and ethnic adult health differences tends to play down the importance of selection processes, when they are recognized at all. The exceptions are few (Adams et al., 2003; Fox et al., 1985; Goldman, 2001; Palloni and Morenoff, 2001; Power et al., 1986; Smith, 1999; West, 1991). The potential damage from such neglect of selection processes could be large and significant (Adams et al., 2003; Ewbank and Jones, 2001; Goldman, 2001; Jasso et al., 2004; Palloni and Ewbank, 2004; Palloni and Morenoff, 2001; Smith, 1999). The stronger the association between prior health status and membership in a group, the larger will be the selection effects. The larger the intergroup difference in the variance of unmeasured traits affecting mortality or health status, the larger will be the influence of heterogeneity. Selection effects may also wane, remain invariant, or increase over time, considerably complicating interpretations of trends in health differences (Goldman, 2001; Vaupel and Yashin, 1985).

To deal with selection processes, one has to avoid treating them simply as nuisances or threats to the validity of a study. Instead, they should be considered part of the reality under investigation. Models that represent the relationships of interest should incorporate selection processes to the extent possible. There are a number of ways of doing this (Palloni and Ewbank, 2004), though in most cases there are strong data requirements and stiff constraints on the inferences that one can draw. Nevertheless, researchers should at least be able to set bounds on the uncertainty surrounding inferences and conclusions.

NEEDED RESEARCH

Selection processes could create or exaggerate differences, or they could offset or disguise them. Identifying and analytically accounting for selection effects (and reciprocal causation) is a substantial, continuing, task. Researchers should either adopt strategies that attenuate some of the associated distortions or, at least, qualify the inferences likely to be drawn. But first they need to recognize the problem and define its reach. Research on health differences in old age should consistently consider the possible operation of selection processes. In most cases, a model representing the genesis of health and mortality differences should include a proper representation of selection processes. To understand and better model selection, research directed at this issue is also advisable.

Research Need 4: Identify and quantify the various selection processes that affect health differences among racial and ethnic groups.

The key reason for the neglect or superficial treatment of selection is the lack of information about the processes underlying it. What data and how much of it should be collected depend on the pertinent selection processes and on the availability of alternative procedures to account for their influence. A good example of the additional information that can be collected involves immigrant surveys that follow individuals from their places of origin to their destinations and through the assimilation process, tracking changes in health, socioeconomic and political status, and other factors (Jasso et al., 2004). (Other suggestions about alternative data collection strategies to account for immigration selection are given by Palloni and Morenoff [2001].)

In particular cases, the data needed could be obtained through modifications of conventional study designs to promote a broader range of comparisons. To understand immigrant selection, for instance, one needs to be able to compare movers and stayers in the origin population, possibly even comparing migrants with siblings, relatives, or in-laws. A transnational study design, though it involves logistical and financial obstacles, is therefore far more useful than a study design based only on the receiving population.

With appropriate data, models could be formulated to yield ranges of estimates for differences as well as confidence intervals. A number of estimation procedures do exist for dealing with a reduced class of selection processes. These should be deployed judiciously, if not to adjust estimates of differences to account for selection processes, at least to provide an idea of the sensitivity of these estimates to assumptions about selection. It is always better to supply information about uncertainty, even if this blurs the scientific conclusions, than to convey the impression of robustness while ignoring potentially relevant effects.

Models should be specifically formulated to allow selection factors to vary in their effects over time. Extant models allow for unmeasured traits to affect selection, but they rest on the rather unyielding and excessively restrictive assumption that these traits and their effects are time-invariant. Fixed traits are surely important, but they may be only a small subset of the relevant factors for health and mortality differences. Since little is known about the magnitude of errors caused by deviations from the assumption of invariance, it is difficult to evaluate whether choosing an incorrect model for selection may lead to more serious problems than ignoring it altogether. More research is needed on the nature, advantages, and shortcomings of models with time-varying effects (Weitz and Fraser, 2001).

3

Genetic Influences

The involvement of genetic factors in racial and ethnic differences in health and disease is currently the focus of intense scrutiny. There are numerous dimensions to this issue. Some have questioned the utility or meaningfulness of the race concept in addressing health issues (e.g., Wilson et al., 2001). Editors have echoed this concern (Anon., 2000, 2001; Schwartz, 2001) and required that submitted manuscripts explain and justify the study of particular ethnic groups or populations (Anon., 2000). At the same time, other researchers report that conventionally defined racial groups differ in genetic factors that affect risk for specific diseases or sensitivity to therapeutic drugs (e.g., Exner et al., 2001; Karter et al., 2002; Splawski et al., 2002; Taioli et al., 1995). Still others have presented the case that racial categories may have biological meaning (Crow, 2002) and can be valuable in biomedical research (Risch et al., 2002).

RACE IN GENETIC PERSPECTIVE

The term race is used in a great variety of ways. Common usage may differ from that of policy makers, and scholarly usage may also vary considerably. Genetic conceptualizations of race, in particular, make reference to differences between and among populations in gene frequencies. The subdiscipline of population genetics is explicitly concerned with such differences and with the dynamics of processes, such as mutation, differential survival, the reproduction of particular gene variants, gene flows between populations through migration, and similar matters. The models for con-

46

ceptualizing and describing these dynamics are highly developed and are clearly central to the taxonomy of human beings.

A key concept is that of genetic distance, of which several measures have been proposed. Basic to these is the probability that a randomly selected allele (see below) from one population will be identical to another allele from the same population but not to one chosen from a different population (see, e.g., Hartl and Clark, 1997). Measures of distance provide metrics that can be used to decide if groups differ sufficiently to be regarded as separate races. But different criteria may be used with respect to how large the genetic distance must be to constitute a racial divide. Some racial classification schemes, therefore, feature many races with small interracial differences, and others identify only a few larger and more separated groups. Each scheme serves its own purposes, and no classification can be regarded as necessarily more correct than others.

In any scheme, the idea of racial identity is a probabilistic one. Different groups are not delineated by clear and unambiguous borders but shade into each other along gradients. Strict categories, exclusive and exhaustive, in which each human being is assignable without ambiguity to one and only one race on the basis of genetic characteristics, are unattainable. Thus, genetics cannot provide a single, definitive human classification scheme with which to address the many facets of health differences.

At the same time, race, as it is socially and politically defined, is a powerful social and political reality. Thus, it is worth asking whether there are identifiable gene differences among socially defined populations or racial groups. The answer to this question requires a distinction between the concepts of genetic loci and genetic alleles. The term locus had its origin at a stage of genetic science when it became evident that the hypothetical elements of Mendelian theory had a physical existence and were located at particular sites, or loci, on chromosomes. A basic postulate of Mendelian theory was that these hypothetical elements (later to be termed genes) could exist in different forms, which came to be termed alleles. Thus, a key question is whether socially defined populations differ in the number or types of loci they possess.

Although it is difficult to prove a universal negative, the evidence is persuasive that all humans possess the same array of genetic loci. The genetic differences among people as individuals consist in the particular array of alleles at these loci; the genetic differences between or among populations can be described in terms of the relative frequencies of the different alleles in the populations. Decades of research in population genetics have documented differences among populations in allelic frequencies for a large number of genetic loci, including many that are health- or disease-related. Of greatest salience for our present topic is the additional observation that the range of genetic differences among individuals within populations usually exceeds by far that between groups. For instance, Hartl and Clark (1997) present an analysis of data from Nei (1975) with respect to a group of enzyme variants, showing that only about 7 percent of the total genetic variation of Caucasoid, Negroid, and Mongoloid racial groups could be assigned to differences among the groups; 93 percent of the variation was within groups. The important consequence is that membership in a particular socially defined race is not a reliable or unambiguous marker for possession of any particular allele (except, perhaps, for such characteristics as skin color).

The Nature of Genetic Influence

The literature also presents a picture of great complexity in the relationships of genes to racial and ethnic health differences. First, it is essential to understand that genetic influence is mediated through a causal nexus comprising the anatomy, biochemistry, physiology, immunology, endocrinology—all of the complex of structures and functions—of the human organism. This is, of course, the same causal nexus through which environmental influences are mediated.

Such complex causal networks are usually characterized by converging and diverging processes derived from multiple inputs from both genetic sources and environmental sources. Multiple redundant pathways with feedback loops may provide for compensatory mechanisms, in which one pathway adjusts for inadequacies in another pathway. Consequences of differences or changes in one of the input elements can be enormously influenced by both genetic and environmental context. The dynamics of these complex causal nexuses underlying health and disease phenotypes is frequently manifest as interactions of genes with genes, genes with environments, or environments with environments.

The resulting causal field is not homogeneous, of course. Some of the inputs and some of the mediating pathways may have a greater impact than others. Some genetic and some environmental variables are sufficiently potent that their influence is apparent in all or most system contexts. In systems terms, there may be nodes within the network that are describable as having a broad "span of control" (Simon, 1973) or as being "soft spots" (Waddington, 1977). In genetic parlance, a gene providing input to a node of this kind may be referred to as a major gene, or a Mendelian gene, or, recklessly, as "the gene" for this or that phenotype. Even the effects of such a major gene, however, may be subject to fine tuning by its companion genes or by the environmental milieu in which all of them operate. Some long-recognized genetic phenomena represent such effects: variable expressivity, in which individuals with the same genotype at a particular locus display different levels of the phenotype associated with the locus; incomplete penetrance, such that some individuals with the genotype do not show the phenotype at all; and variable time of onset, in which individuals with the same disease genotype vary widely in the age at which symptoms appear.

In respect to health and disease, genetic loci for which particular allelic configurations result with high reliability in a diagnosable disease outcome are often described as "disease genes." However, particular genotypes at other genetic loci may affect the same general categorical disease state. Thus, many disease genes, though they may be sufficient, are not necessary for the expression of the disease phenotype. In other cases, as in the association between the ε4 allele of the *apoE* locus and Alzheimer's disease (discussed below), the identified allele is neither necessary nor sufficient. In different populations, the same disease state may be achieved by different genotypes affecting different mediating mechanisms.

Other disease states may not be categorically distinct from the normal range of variability of some anatomic structure or physiological process but may constitute extremes of such a dimension. The location of an individual in continuously distributed phenotypes is typically due to the action of many genetic loci, as well as many environmental variables. Any particular value of such a continuously distributed phenotype can be achieved by numerous combinations of input variables. The genetic input is described as polygenic. Analysis of such systems is generally statistical, with a central theme being the attribution of proportions of the measured phenotypic variability into two broad categories, genetic and environmental, and, depending on the research design, into more detailed categories, such as additive or nonadditive genetic effects and shared or nonshared environmental influences.

Gene Interactions

In considering ethnic identity and health, genes may be relevant in two broad senses. First, the gene pools of different ethnic groups may contain different frequencies of alleles at some loci that are pertinent to health status or to disease processes. However, such differences by themselves are unlikely to account for broad and pervasive health differences among socially identified racial and ethnic groups.

Second, the phenotype consequent on a given genotype may vary between ethnic groups because of interactions with environmental factors. The environment, in this context, is defined by exclusion, as all influences not coded in DNA. It thus covers all the other factors noted in Chapter 2, including prenatal effects, nutritional influences, the preventive consequences of health care, peer group pressures, educational level, religious instruction, toxins in homes and in the air and water, occupational hazards, job stress, and exposure to infectious agents, among many, many others.

Much is known about the etiological significance of a vast array of such environmental factors; much also is known about the influence of major genes and of polygenic systems. Conceptually, the possibility of interactions within and between these two broad domains has long been recognized. For various reasons, research emphasizing and characterizing these interactions has been less well developed than might be expected. Their implications for health differences are not yet known, though the accumulated literature, both from human and animal model research, is substantial. Only a few examples are cited here, but they should illustrate the great complexity and power and the sometimes astonishing subtlety of these interactions.

In human beings, interaction between two major genes is implicated in the etiology of the large and burgeoning health problem of Alzheimer's disease. Three different alleles—$\varepsilon 2$, $\varepsilon 3$, and $\varepsilon 4$—have been described at the *apoE* locus on chromosome 19. In general, possession of one $\varepsilon 4$ allele is associated with an increased risk of developing Alzheimer's disease, and possession of two confers a greater risk than possession of one. This latter outcome, however, depends on the genotype at another locus, *ACT*. In the case of one genotype at that locus, there is no difference in risk of having one or two $\varepsilon 4$ alleles at the *apoE* locus; for another *ACT* genotype, the risk is somewhat elevated; and for the third, the difference in risk between one and two $\varepsilon 4$ alleles is fivefold. Clearly, when considering differences in allelic frequency in different populations, it may be necessary to be concerned with dyads, triads, or larger collectives of loci.

A classic animal model study showing that the effect of different genotypes at a major locus can be modified by the polygenic background of the organism is the work of Coleman and Hummel (1975). Two copies of a particular allele at a specific locus generally lead to some manifestation of diabetes in mice, but in two different but related strains the resulting syndromes are strikingly different, with blood glucose levels and body weight differing twofold, large differences in lifespans, and Islet hypertrophy in one strain and atrophy in the other.

Perhaps the prototypic illustration of interaction between polygenes and the environment is that of Cooper and Zubek (1958), who measured the maze learning ability of two lines of rats reared under environmental conditions that differed in the variety of stimuli that the animals could experience. The two strains had been selectively bred for maze performance (Heron, 1935); the resulting "maze-bright" and "maze-dull" lines differed strikingly in the number of errors committed in learning the maze pattern, and, by strong inference, in terms of allelic configurations at an unknown number of polygenic loci pertinent to maze performance. The results of differential rearing were that the bright lines did not profit from enrichment, but the dull ones did; the dull rats were not adversely affected by impoverishment, but the bright ones were. Numerous other studies have shown similar differential responses in a variety of phenotypes to environmental manipulations by groups of mice or rats of differing genotypes.

Another striking recent example of gene-environment interaction is provided by the study of quantitative trait loci (QTLs) affecting longevity in *Drosophila* flies. QTLs are loci that remain anonymous at present, but whose approximate chromosomal locations are known. Vieira et al. (2000) sought evidence for the effect of such loci on the length of life under five different environmental conditions of rearing. The extraordinary result was that 17 QTLs were identified, but none was pertinent to all environments. Some were effective in one sex only and in one environment; others were effective in both sexes in a specific environment, but the same allele was associated with longer lives in one sex and shorter lives in the other sex; some were effective in one sex in two environments, but with the same allele associated with longer lives in one environment and shorter lives in the other. All of the genetic variance was involved in genotype x sex interactions, genotype x environment interactions, or both.

Within the general domain of coaction of genes and environmental factors, there are several lines of investigation that convincingly demonstrate that environments not only can interact in a statistical sense with genetic factors, but can also actually influence which genes are expressed. In an oversimplified explanation, some environments can turn genes on and off. Certain subdomains of this research are of particular potential relevance for the present topic, dealing with the effects of stress of various sorts on gene expression. For instance, an extensive body of literature (summarized, for example, by Hoffman and Parsons, 1991) describes observations that suggest that stressful environments often increase the heritability—the proportion of phenotypic variance attributable to the collective influence of a polygenic system—of a wide variety of phenotypes in a wide array of organisms. A major body of data dealing with specific genes concerns the "heat-shock" proteins that are produced in *Drosophila* after exposure to a high-temperature environment. These proteins appear to protect other proteins in the organism from damage or destruction by the stressful environment. An example from mammals is the increase in the levels of specific RNAs in the adrenal glands of rats following immobilization stress (McMahon et al., 1992). Biobehavioral influences are clearly implicated by a study showing that classical Pavlovian conditioning—pairing foot-shock and an auditory stimulus—can result in a previously neutral feature of the environment acquiring the capability of eliciting a stress-related expression of a particular mRNA in regions of the brain of rats (Smith et al., 1992). These lines of research are perhaps particularly relevant to hypotheses concerning the role of discrimination stress, such as those of Thayer and Friedman (2004).

Some Racial and Ethnic Differences

These various studies offer conceptual lenses for considering evidence of genetic influences on ethnic differences in health and disease. Several recent examples illustrate the pertinent evidence being presented.

Differential responsiveness to therapy has been identified by Exner et al. (2001), who compared black and white patients with left ventricular dysfunction on response to Enalapril therapy. Briefly, black patients displayed no significant reduction of risk for hospitalization for heart failure within 36 months of therapy, while white patients experienced a 44 percent reduction in risk. Other such racial differences have been identified, such as greater resistance among black kidney and liver transplant patients to immunosuppression (Nagashima et al., 2001). The mechanisms underlying these physiological differences may, of course, be environmental, genetic, or some combination of these effects.

Research that more explicitly implicates genetic factors can be illustrated by that of Splawski et al. (2002), who found a particular allele (described as Y1102) of a gene (SCN5A) to be associated with arrhythmia in blacks. This allele is found in about 13 percent of blacks and in about 19 percent of West Africans and Caribbeans, but it has not yet been identified in whites or Asians. Y1102 increases the risk of arrhythmia but is not a sufficient cause—most carriers of the allele never display arrhythmia. The conjecture is that the gene operates in the context of other risk factors, including possibly the use of certain medications.

A further example is provided by Karter et al. (2002), who examined the complications experienced by diabetics who participated in the same medical care program. The results differed by type of complication: blacks, Asians, and Hispanics had a substantially lower incidence of myocardial infarction than did whites; blacks experienced more strokes than whites; Asians had many fewer lower extremity amputations; and whites had lower incidence of end-stage renal disease. Complication susceptibility is clearly not the exclusive attribute of any one group.

Contextual scrutiny of genetic factors thus can lead to discoveries of important gene-gene and gene-environment interactions. For instance, there is evidence that the apoE genotype is less of a risk factor in Hispanic or black populations than in Caucasian populations (Sahota et al., 1997). Whether these differences are due to gene-gene interactions, gene-environment interactions, or both remains to be demonstrated.

Increasingly, reference is made to the prospects of individualized medicine, in which the preventive or intervention strategies will be tailored to the relevant genotype of the individuals. The foregoing discussion about interactions has emphasized that it will be necessary for the genotypic information to be joined with environmental information. The identification of all of the relevant input variables for all health and disease issues will be a formidable undertaking. Fortunately, benefits will be derived from the partial knowledge that will be generated on the way. Increasingly, it will be possible for medical decisions to be informed by information about DNA as well as about environmental circumstances of the individual. Racial identity, at best a weak surrogate for these genetic and environmental factors, will become increasingly irrelevant in treatment of disease.

NEEDED RESEARCH

In broad terms, both genetic and environmental factors, particularly in interaction, play a role in racial and ethnic differences in health and disease. These factors are active subjects of investigation by the genetic and social sciences separately.

Research Need 5: Assess genetic and environmental factors in racial and ethnic differences in health simultaneously, in designs that permit identification of both main effects and interactions.

This research focus necessarily would emphasize the identification and assessment of environmental features, both physical and sociocultural, that are pertinent to ethnic differences in health outcomes. The range of environmental variables should be considered in a life-course perspective, with attention to the possibility of the existence of critical periods for environmental impact. Attractive research opportunities are offered by populations of particular ethnic groups in similar settings and life circumstances.

The potential value of concentration of research efforts on interactions is self-evident. If the incidence or severity of a disease related to a particular genotype is dependent on the environment, detailed examination of the mechanism through which environmental influence is mediated may suggest preventive as well as ameliorative measures. The advantages would accrue to individuals of all racial and ethnic groups.

Genetic comparisons among populations of course need to continue. Characterization of gene frequency differences among populations should be strongly oriented toward the detection of epistatic (interactive) gene networks, and the newly available molecular procedures for identifying and characterizing genes and evaluating the level of gene expression should be melded with quantitative methods for dealing with complex phenotypes.

As in all domains of biomedical research, although human beings are our targeted concern, some aspects of complex systems are most efficiently approached through animal models.

4

Socioeconomic Status

A considerable body of evidence has established that individuals of low socioeconomic status are more likely to suffer from disease, to experience loss of functioning, to be cognitively and physically impaired, and to experience higher mortality (Adler et al., 1993, 1994; Marmot et al., 1997b; Preston and Taubman, 1994; Rogers et al., 2000; Williams, 1990). As illustrated in Figure 4-1, this association holds true for nearly all major causes of morbidity, functioning loss, disability, and mortality. This figure uses education as an indicator of socioeconomic status; similar data using income, occupation, or wealth would generally show the same relationships. For instance, Table 4-1 shows that a similar relationship between wealth and self-reported health holds across adult ages.

THE HEALTH GRADIENT AND RECIPROCAL CAUSATION

The influence of socioeconomic status on health is assumed to begin in the prenatal environment and continue through life. Parents' socioeconomic status affects childhood conditions, such as exposure to toxins and infectious agents. These conditions affect health immediately and possibly for years afterwards, the effects being only partly moderated by later changes in status (Blackwell et al., 2000; Hayward et al., 2000; Kuh and Davey-Smith, 1997; Preston et al., 1998). Childhood socioeconomic differences have been recently shown to account for a substantial part of the later mortality gap between blacks and whites (Warner and Hayward, 2002).

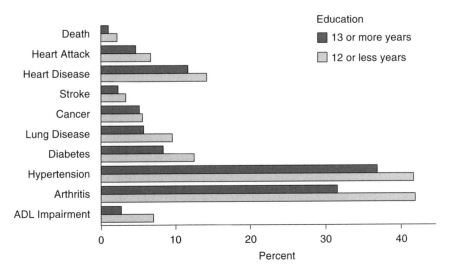

FIGURE 4-1 Death within 2 years and prevalence of various conditions, by years of education (in percent).
NOTE: ADL, activities of daily life.
SOURCE: Data from Health and Retirement Survey, as reported by Crimmins et al. (2004).

The health gradient by socioeconomic status widens through childhood and the adult working years and then contracts after retirement (Case et al., 2002; Crimmins et al., 2004; House et al., 1994). After some age, changes in some aspects of socioeconomic status have diminishing effects on health; it is unclear which changes in aspects of socioeconomic status continue to affect health in old age.

Assessing the effect of lifetime socioeconomic conditions on health is complicated by the fact that health also affects income and wealth, especially among adults (Smith, 1999). Table 4-1 shows that those with "fair" or "poor" self-reported health in 1984 not only had much lower wealth in that year but also saw their wealth grow less than that of others over the next 10 years. Though the table does not show it, smaller gains in wealth were associated with less favorable health outcomes.

Reciprocal causation has been one of the most difficult issues to deal with in this literature, and it is often ignored or dismissed as a minor factor. However, Smith and Kington (1997) show that much of the correlation between current income and health among males in their 50s appears to be the effect of health on income, rather than the reverse, and Adams et al. (2003) argue that among the retired population, there may be no income

TABLE 4-1 Median Household Wealth and Self-Reported Health Status

Age Group and 1984 Health Status	Wealth (in thousands)[a]		
	1984	1989	1994
All Households			
Excellent	68.3	99.3	127.9
Very good	66.3	81.9	90.9
Good	51.8	59.6	64.9
Fair/poor	39.2	36.0	34.7
25-34			
Excellent	28.5	51.5	84.3
Very good	19.5	34.7	50.1
Good	10.5	17.2	28.2
Fair/poor	0.9	3.1	10.4
35-44			
Excellent	100.1	150.1	194.7
Very good	81.1	96.3	117.5
Good	49.5	45.3	83.5
Fair/poor	23.8	15.5	32.4
45-54			
Excellent	164.2	198.3	255.8
Very good	132.1	176.2	186.9
Good	87.8	76.9	97.1
Fair/poor	59.7	61.6	69.4

[a]In 1996 dollars.
SOURCE: Data from Panel Study of Income Dynamics, as reported by Smith (1999: Table 1, p. 147).

effects on health. The key question is not which of the two alternative pathways can be dismissed entirely. Rather, the more appropriate question may be which subset of the well-documented associations between socioeconomic status and health is most susceptible to interpretations that flow from health to status.

STATUS, RACE, AND ETHNICITY

The health gradient by socioeconomic status is important for racial and ethnic differences because socioeconomic status differs considerably by race and ethnicity. Table 4-2 shows some variations in socioeconomic status among older people. Older black and Hispanics are much less likely than whites to have a high school diploma or a college degree and much more likely to live in poverty. Older Asians have relatively more education, but compared with whites, twice the percentage of them live in poverty. Similar figures for American Indians and Alaska Natives are not available, but

TABLE 4-2 Socioeconomic Status by Race and Ethnicity Among Persons
Aged 65 Years and Older

Racial or Ethnic Group	Percentage with		Percentage in Poverty		
	High School Diploma 1998	Bachelor's Degree 1998	Both Sexes 1998	Men 1997	Women 1997
White	71.6	16.0	8.2	5.6	11.5
Black	43.7	7.0	26.4	21.8	28.8
Hispanic	29.4	5.4	21.0	20.3	26.3
Asian or Pacific Islander	65.1	22.2	16.0	— [a]	— [a]

[a]No data.
SOURCES: Data from Federal Interagency Forum on Aging Related Statistics (2000) and
Kramarow et al. (1999).

1990 household data suggest levels of poverty among American Indians
similar to those for blacks, and levels for Alaska Natives similar to those for
Asians (U.S. Census Bureau, 1990). Socioeconomic variations such as these,
coupled with similar variations at younger ages, partly explain racial and
ethnic differences in a number of health outcomes (Hayward et al., 2000;
Smith and Kington, 1997).

When socioeconomic status is controlled, health differences between
blacks and whites in mortality and functional limitations are sometimes
eliminated (Kington and Smith, 1997), though differences may not disappear for specific diseases. Good examples of large racial or ethnic differences that are not explained by socioeconomic status are hypertension
among black men and diabetes among black and Hispanic men (Crimmins
et al., 2004). There also appear to be significant nonlinearities in the effects
of income and wealth, as these factors have a much stronger effect on
health in the bottom third of their respective distributions than in the top
third. Taking these nonlinearities into account may help further explain
black-white health differences. However, the role of socioeconomic status
in explaining Asian-white differences is less clear, and it does not explain
the relative health advantage of Hispanics.

One complication in any comparison is the possibility that socioeconomic measures may signify something different for each group (Kaufman
et al., 1997; Williams and Collins, 1995). Black high school graduates, for
instance, do not exhibit the same levels of knowledge and skills as whites
(Maxwell, 1994). Equal incomes may not be truly equal if they do not
translate into the same purchasing power in different communities (Alexis
et al., 1980; Williams and Collins, 1995). The effect on health differences if

controls were possible with exactly equivalent socioeconomic measures is not known.

MECHANISMS

Socioeconomic status affects health through a variety of mechanisms, including psychosocial factors, health behaviors, and health care (Anderson, 1995; Hummer et al., 1998; Kington and Nickens, 2001; Seeman and Crimmins, 2001). In general, persons of higher socioeconomic status are less exposed to health-threatening conditions and have more resources to buffer health threats. For instance, persons with more education have greater ability to self-monitor and manage highly effective but complicated therapies for such conditions as diabetes and HIV (Goldman and Smith, 2002). Variation in this ability may involve other factors in addition to education, however. In general, the intervening mechanisms that have been studied through which socioeconomic status affects health—such as behavior risk factors (Lantz et al., 2001)—do not entirely account for the effects of socioeconomic status, leaving much of these effects still to be explained. In addition, these intervening mechanisms could operate independently of socioeconomic status.

Additional factors may also obscure the effects of status. For instance, recent immigrants often have lower incomes, at least initially, but enjoy health advantages for other reasons. Working-age immigrants, particularly those with employment visas or who enter as spouses of U.S. citizens, appear to be strongly selected for health (Jasso et al., 2004). Assessing the role of socioeconomic factors in group health, therefore, requires attention to health in countries of origin and to the average healthiness of the original immigrants, the diversity in health status among them, and their subsequent health trajectories over their lifetimes and those of their descendants.

In addition to these individual-level mechanisms, considerable research in the last decade argues that macrolevel socioeconomic factors affect individual health outcomes (Marmot, 2000; Wilkinson, 1997). One form of the hypothesis is that inequality, as measured in various ways, has a negative effect on individual health outcomes, especially for those at the bottom of the social and economic hierarchy. In this view, the cumulative stress of being at the bottom of the hierarchy eventually takes a toll in poorer health. This is an important scientific hypothesis with far-reaching implications. However, much of the influential early work on this subject suffered from severe limitations, including inadequate conceptualization of and difficulties in separating individual from macrolevel influences. Recent work by Deaton and Paxson (2001) argues that, at least for U.S. blacks and whites, the evidence that rising levels of income inequality have negative health consequences is dubious.

Another factor strongly linked to socioeconomic status is the quality of one's physical environment (Adler and Newman, 2002; Evans and Kantrowitz, 2002). U.S. data indicate that substandard housing, crowding, elevated noise levels, limited ability to regulate temperature and humidity, and exposure to noxious pollutants and allergens (including lead, smog, particulates, and dust mites) are all common in poor, segregated communities (Been, 1997; Bullard, 1994; Evans and Saegert, 2000; Mohai and Bryant, 1992, 1998; Pearlin et al., 2001). For both adults and children, increased respiratory and other health problems result from residing near hazardous waste sites (Dolk et al., 1998; Goldberg et al., 1999), residential exposure to air pollution (Keeler et al., 2002; Pope et al., 2002; Thurston and Ito, 2001), and deteriorated housing conditions (Peat et al., 1998; Rauh et al., 2002). However, the exact contribution of such environmental conditions to racial and ethnic differences in health status, and the extent to which they add to other socioeconomic effects or possibly explain them, is still unclear.

NEEDED RESEARCH

Although socioeconomic status is strongly linked to health, many research questions remain about the nature of this linkage and the contribution of socioeconomic status to racial and ethnic health differences.

Research Need 6: Clarify the degree to which socioeconomic status accounts for racial and ethnic differences in health outcomes over the life course.

Some differences are not explained by socioeconomic status, or even run counter to the expected. Would better measures of education, or other aspects of status, provide clarification? Would incorporating measures of earlier socioeconomic status, perhaps status prior to immigration, explain more of the differences? Is better modeling needed of presumed nonlinear relationships? What differences in health outcomes would still not be explained even if all these questions could be answered? The possibility that the effects of socioeconomic factors are misestimated because of differential survival by race and ethnic group also requires consideration.

One complication is that dimensions of socioeconomic status are not identical in their effects on racial and ethnic health differences. Analysts need to know the most appropriate aspect of status to consider—income, wealth, education, or occupation. Health differences by race or ethnicity will look different if one or the other indicator is controlled. Policy makers need to know which aspect of status matters most. It makes a great deal of difference to policy whether differences are largely due to income, in which case increasing the income of the poor gains greater weight from its possible effect on health; or education, in which case equality of educational opportunity, or affecting the outcomes of education—improving individual access to information and the ability to process it effectively—become long-term priorities. That identical levels on the same indicators may have different implications across groups also requires attention.

Variability in the effect of socioeconomic status over the life course is an additional complication. In late life, which aspects of status have the most influence on health? At the start of the life course, socioeconomic status is acquired from one's parents, who not only provide financial support but also influence the education of their children. Children may also acquire from their parents habits and personal characteristics that directly affect health. How intergenerational transmission of all these factors is patterned by race or ethnicity may be important, given the influence of early life factors on late-life health. Reciprocal causation between socioeconomic status and health is an important aspect of the lifelong effect of status, and whether it operates similarly across the life course for different racial and ethnic groups needs study.

Research Need 7: Identify the mechanisms through which socioeconomic status produces racial and ethnic differences in health among the elderly, and identify other factors that complicate its effects.

Socioeconomic status may have an effect because of its links to commonly recognized health behaviors, other psychosocial factors, multiple dimensions of access to health care, geographic residence, environmental conditions, and nativity and duration of residence, especially for Hispanics and other immigrant groups. In what circumstances, or for which subgroups, are racial and ethnic differences robust to controls for such variables? Which controls are most important and why? If none of them adequately explain the effects of status, how does it come to modify health outcomes?

This analysis will require attending not just to socioeconomic variation in disease prevalence but to variation in the disease process: the onset of conditions, their severity, duration, and effects on survival (Crimmins et al., 2004). The relevant mechanisms may differ at each stage.

Whether macrolevel mechanisms are important is another aspect worth studying. Can aggregate effects be verified, and is income inequality the most appropriate aggregate indicator? If such aggregate effects exist, how do they work—at the local, regional, or societal levels, or even at the workplace level, and through what mechanisms? How are such aggregate macromarkers related to other aggregate variables, such as social capital and group cohesion, and how do such factors vary by race and ethnicity?

5

Behavior Risk Factors

One possible way in which socioeconomic status can become embodied—therefore producing health differences between groups that differ in status—is through producing variation in behavior risk factors—in smoking, over-eating, not exercising, and other such behaviors. We consider these behavior risk factors here, but leave for later, for the health care section, such other behaviors as health care seeking and patient compliance.

BEHAVIORAL VARIATION

Some behavior risk factors clearly affect health in late life, as a variety of studies show. For instance, Østbye et al. (2002) looked longitudinally at the effects of various behaviors on a variety of health outcomes, including inability to work, dependence on others in activities of daily living, self-reported health status, and hospitalization. For middle-aged and older Americans, smoking was consistently related to ill health however measured, as was lack of exercise and obesity (though a very low body mass index, or BMI, also increased risk) and past problems with alcohol (see also, e.g., Allison et al., 1997; Burke et al., 2001; Davis et al., 1994; Launer et al., 1994; Stuck et al., 1999; Thun et al., 1997). These behaviors are among the major risk factors associated with heart disease, cancer, and other morbidities (McGinnis and Foege, 1993). They appear to explain part—though generally a small part—of variation by education and income in functional and self-rated health and disease (Crimmins et al., 2004; Lantz et al., 2001).

A few studies suggest age limits to the effects of some behavior risk factors. Perhaps beyond age 70 or so, those who are still healthy may be less affected by continuing to smoke or being overweight (Crimmins, 2001; Seeman et al., 1994; Strawbridge et al., 1996). Other studies, however, show continued effects at advanced ages (Reed et al., 1998). Previous behavior, at younger ages, could, in particular cases, be of diminishing relevance. This effect has been demonstrated for smoking: people who quit smoking by their mid-40s show no adverse effects by their late 50s, if they survive to that age, relative to those who never smoked (Østbye et al., 2002; Peto et al., 2000). More generally, however, behavior earlier in life predicts later behavior and may have long-term effects not fully accounted for (Warner and Hayward, 2002).

Racial and ethnic groups differ on these behaviors (Bolen et al., 2000; Schoenborn and Barnes, 2002); see Table 5-1. Relative to whites, American Indians and Alaska Natives exhibit less healthy behaviors, and Asians generally healthier behaviors, except in having less leisure-time physical activity. Blacks and Hispanics also have less leisure-time physical activity than whites, and both these groups are more likely to be obese, though the contrast is less sharp for Hispanics. In addition, Hispanics report slightly more binge drinking than whites, but blacks report sharply less. (Drinking patterns are complex, however, showing cultural patterning across nationality groups that persists across generations [Dawson, 1998].)

These risk behaviors may not be independently chosen but may represent a syndrome of risk affinity or aversion. Counting the number of behavior risk factors—and adding such preventive behaviors as colorectal screening—Hahn et al. (2000) confirm that American Indians and Alaska Natives and blacks have a significantly larger number of behavior risk factors than whites, and Asians a significantly smaller number, even controlling for socioeconomic factors.

Men and women are not distinguished in Table 5-1, but gender differences could be important (Winkleby and Cubbin, 2004). If one looks specifically at men and women aged 65-74, the picture becomes more complicated, particularly for blacks. Higher levels of obesity and inactivity, relative to whites, appear mainly for older black women, but not for older black men. And cigarette smoking does appear relatively more common among older black men relative to whites, though not among younger black men nor among black women of any age (Sundquist et al., 2001; Winkleby and Cubbin, 2004).

REASONS FOR VARIATION

Socioeconomic disadvantage is one reason for differences in behavior risk factors. Less education, for instance, is associated with more smoking

TABLE 5-1 Self-Reported Health Risk Behaviors, by Race and Ethnicity

Behavior	White	Black	Hispanic	Asian	American Indian/ Alaska Native
Current Cigarette Smoking					
Median percent[a]	23.6	22.8	23.1	10.7	41.3
Percentage of states where group median exceeds white median	—	46.0	47.0	11.0	82.0
States included	—	34	35	9	11
No Leisure-Time Physical Activity in Last 30 Days					
Median percent[a]	25.1	38.2	34.2	28.9	37.2
Percentage of states where group median exceeds white median	—	92.0	81.0	100	100
States included	—	36	35	6	5
Obesity[b]					
Median percent[a]	15.6	26.4	18.2	4.8	30.1
Percentage of states where group median exceeds white median	—	97.0	73.0	20.0	91.0
States included	—	35	35	10	11
Binge Drinking[c]					
Median percent[a]	14.5	8.7	16.2	6.7	18.9
Percentage of states where group median exceeds white median	—	11.0	66.0	25.0	91.0
States included	—	35	35	8	11

[a]Median percentages across states; fewer states are represented for minorities, particularly the last two groups, because of small samples.
[b]Body mass index of 30 kg/m^2 or higher.
[c]Five or more alcoholic drinks at least once in past month.
SOURCE: Data from Behavioral Risk Factor Surveillance System, 1997 (Bolen et al., 2000: Table 24).

and less physical activity, even among high-functioning people aged 70-79 (Kubzansky et al., 1998). Controlling for education and income reduces the apparent behavioral disadvantages of blacks and Hispanics at all adult ages. However, it does not increase any advantage in lower alcohol consumption, and one marginal difference—a Hispanic advantage in lower cigarette smoking—becomes significant when socioeconomic factors are taken into account (Winkleby and Cubbin, 2004). Some differences clearly cannot be explained by socioeconomic factors, at least to the extent socioeconomic differences can presently be measured (Braveman et al., 2001; Kaufman et al., 1997). Whether controlling for home ownership and other assets would eliminate more of the behavioral differences is not known. Even adding such controls in one study, however, leaves untouched a large part of the black disadvantage, relative to whites, in cardiovascular disease indicators (Rooks et al., 2002).

Another source of behavioral differences may be cultural, or more specifically, degree of acculturation among immigrants and their descendants (Espino et al., 1991; Jasso et al., 2000). The more acculturated a person—whether Hispanic, Asian, or black—the more prone the person is to smoking and obesity, whether acculturation is determined from United States versus foreign birth, duration of residence in the United States, or language spoken at home (Singh and Siahpush, 2002; Winkleby and Cubbin, 2004). Various cultural beliefs, such as the presumed attractiveness of moderately overweight women, have also been proposed as important (Stevens et al., 1994).

An additional factor that may produce behavioral differences is the residential environment. Neighborhoods provide stimuli, such as outlets for alcohol or illegal drugs, or limit options for healthy nutrition or exercise. Black neighborhoods appear more likely to suffer from such institutional risk factors as the proliferation of liquor stores and insufficient supplies of prescription drugs (LaVeist and Wallace, 2000; Morrison et al., 2000). However, since blacks have lower rates of drinking and smoking than whites—an advantage that increases when socioeconomic status is controlled—the implications of such neighborhood disadvantages are unclear. Differences do indeed appear across neighborhoods in smoking, dietary practices, physical activity, and substance abuse (Morenoff and Lynch, 2004; Winkleby and Cubbin, 2004). Whether these are due mainly to socioeconomic deprivation in poorer neighborhoods or actually reflect some effect of the neighborhood environment is difficult to verify.

EFFECTS OF VARIATION AND TRENDS

Does variation in these behavior risk factors account for some portion of racial and ethnic differences in health? This issue has been insufficiently studied, especially for comparisons other than black and white. Behavioral factors clearly do not explain all differences, and how much they do explain is unclear.

Looking at black-white differences in mortality, Otten et al. (1990) combined behavior risk factors (smoking, BMI, and alcohol intake) and some health outcomes closely linked to behavior (systolic blood pressure, cholesterol level, and diabetes). Among persons 35-54 years old, those factors combined explained 31 percent of the excess mortality for blacks relative to whites. Slightly more of the mortality differential was explained by income, while a larger proportion remained unexplained.

With a narrower definition of behavior risk factors, less of the health differences can be accounted for. In a separate analysis of self-reported health among individuals aged 51-61 years (Smith and Kington, 1997), a cluster of behavioral factors—the most important of which was BMI—account for only about one-sixth of the black disadvantage relative to whites, and it did not affect the Hispanic disadvantage. Among individuals aged 70 and older, the effect of behavior risk factors on self-reported health is slightly greater, with the black disadvantage reduced by one-third and the Hispanic disadvantage by close to one-fifth. These results are largely independent of socioeconomic status.

The role of behavior risk factors is even smaller in a study by Warner and Hayward (2002) of a sample of older men. They find that, once socioeconomic and demographic factors are taken into account, behavior factors do not explain the mortality gap. The opposite is true: with socioeconomic and demographic factors controlled, black risk behavior appears more favorable for health than white behavior, mainly because, with socioeconomic status controlled, blacks smoke less.

Such comparisons are mostly confined to black and whites. Given the somewhat contradictory patterns—Hispanics and Asians both having lower mortality rates than whites (but in one case exhibiting generally riskier behavior and in the other case less risky behavior)—it seems unlikely that, whatever the effects of these behaviors, they account for a substantial portion of health differences.

Could the effects of similar behaviors be different across racial and ethnic groups? Systematic study of this question has not been done, though hypotheses to this effect have been offered (e.g., Pampel, 1998). Work on obesity and alcohol consumption may be used to illustrate the possibilities and the uncertainties.

Obesity among older blacks, according to several studies summarized by Stevens (2000), is less of a risk factor for mortality than among whites (see also Sanchez et al., 2000). This differential effect appears mainly to involve black women. Although a dose-response relationship can be shown between BMI (above a minimum BMI of around 23) and mortality rate for whites of either gender, no such effect is visible for black women in several studies (e.g., Calle et al., 1999; Stevens, 2000; Stevens et al., 1998). It has also been suggested that obesity may even have a protective effect among older Hispanics (Stern et al., 1990). There are contradictory studies, however. For instance, Allison et al. (1997) find the same association of BMI with mortality for blacks and whites among men and women 70 years and older. And Grabowski and Ellis (2001) find, for a predominantly white sample of people of the same age, no association of elevated BMI with mortality. Several explanations are possible for such conflicting findings, including restricted samples, the uneven effect of selection, variations in model specification, the confounding relationship of smoking with BMI, and possible differences in the distribution of body fat (Stern et al., 1990). Some generally negative effect of obesity on health—though not necessarily moderate overweight—is likely (Casper, 1995; Rössner, 2001), though attending to ethnicity clearly complicates the issue.

Alcohol consumption may also vary in its effects across racial and ethnic groups. As with BMI, alcohol consumption has a U-shaped or J-shaped relationship to mortality, at least beginning around age 35. The number of drinks associated with minimum mortality risk rises with age (White et al., 2002). Epidemiological studies have also found a minimum for deterioration in cognitive performance, which begins around four to eight drinks a day for men and two to four drinks a day for women (Dufouil et al., 1997; Elias et al., 1999; Kalmijn et al., 2002). For older Japanese Americans in Hawaii, however, cognitive performance declines at lower levels, beginning at about one drink a day (Bond et al., 2001; Galanis et al., 2000). A genetic factor may be involved: the fact that 50 percent of Japanese and Chinese lack the active form of aldehyde hydrogenase (ALDH2) and therefore have a lower alcohol elimination rate (Bond et al., 2001; Eckardt et al., 1998).

Health-related risk behaviors could get worse for groups with large proportions of immigrants. As noted above, acculturation is related to increases in both smoking and obesity, which are initially lower among immigrants than natives. Nor does rising socioeconomic status among minorities always reduce risky behavior. Consider the relationship between obesity and education. Educational levels are rising, from which one might infer the spread of healthier behavior. However, higher education increases physical activity more for whites than blacks, as well as reducing alcohol consumption more among whites (Gallant and Dorn, 2001). Furthermore, within each educational level, obesity is also rising—and it is rising faster among blacks than whites (Himes and Reynolds, 2002). Future generations of the older adults will be made up of individuals whose youthful habits, for whatever environmental and generational reasons, will have been less favorable to maintaining health.

OTHER BEHAVIORS

We have considered major behavior risk factors that affect chronic illness. Other behaviors may also be relevant. Substance abuse and unsafe sex, for instance, may also vary across groups and produce racial and ethnic differences (Anderson, 1995). These behaviors are of greater concern among younger adults, but they are also relevant for older people. In a British sample of people over 50 years old, for instance, 7 percent reported behavior that put them at risk of contracting sexually transmitted diseases (Gott,

2001), a proportion that could conceivably vary by race and ethnicity in the United States, given variation in sexually transmitted diseases by socio-economic status. In addition, behavior at younger ages could have long-term health effects or determine which people survive to older ages. Other behaviors, such as suicide, are more directly relevant to older adults, though suicide may be better addressed as a consequence of such factors as depression (Myers and Hwang, 2004). (Preventive health behaviors are considered below in relation to health care.)

As an illustration of the potential effect on differences of a range of other behavior risk factors, consider such a simple behavior—with complex causes—as staying in one's home versus going out regularly. One case shows how this can produce racial and ethnic differences in mortality. A heat wave in Chicago in July 1995 killed at least 521 and possibly as many as 739 people, mostly older adults (Klinenberg, 2002; Whitman et al., 1997). The age-adjusted black death rate was 50 percent higher than the white rate. Hispanic fatalities were so low that a rate could not be calculated. Those most vulnerable proved to be people who lived alone, did not leave home daily, had medical problems, were confined to bed, and had no air conditioning (Semenza et al., 1996). The ethnic difference had much to do with the quality of neighborhood life. Equally poor black and Hispanic neighborhoods were characterized by relatively empty and unsafe versus bustling streets, and few commercial attractions versus animated public spaces. Overall, a pervasive fear of violence in black neighborhoods kept seniors especially indoors, with disastrous results (Klinenberg, 2002). Other behavioral factors can therefore be highly consequential for health differences, and are tied in to neighborhood features, which may in turn have roots in discrimination and lack of social support, factors that we consider further below.

NEEDED RESEARCH

Much is uncertain about the role of behavior risk factors in racial and ethnic differences, leading to a number of important research issues.

Research Need 8: Study how behavior risk factors act over the life course in different racial and ethnic groups.

The effects of behavior among older adults, in contrast to the effects at younger ages, sometimes appear weaker or nonexistent, and carefully designed studies are needed to avoid such pitfalls as inadequate samples and unrecognized selection effects. Behavior does show some consistency over time, but it can also change. The intricacies of attending to cohort and period changes in such factors as smoking, diet, and exercise, their delayed effects on health outcomes in later years, and the differences in these relationships across racial and ethnic groups provide a substantial challenge to researchers.

The possibility that behavior has different effects for different groups needs broader investigation. Work in this area has focused mainly on obesity among blacks and whites, leading so far to inconclusive findings. If different effects can be confirmed, more work would be needed to investigate the possible reasons. Attention is also needed to other ethnic groups, such as Hispanics, for whom obesity may still be risky but possibly proportionally less of a risk: if this is confirmed, it might shed further light on the mechanisms involved.

Variation in behavior risk factors across racial and ethnic groups cannot be accounted for solely by socioeconomic factors. While other factors have been suggested, especially acculturation, these are probably insufficient to account, for instance, for the relatively unhealthy behaviors among American Indians and Alaska Natives and blacks. Such problematic conditions as obesity among black women need to be better understood. The reasons for the high rates, and the reasons that obesity sometimes appears to have proportionally less effect than in other groups, need to be clarified. Cutler et al. (2003) argue that overweight and obesity have increased most among those, often women, who have benefited most from technological innovations that have made foods more convenient and reduced food preparation effort. Whether this argument has anything to do with the obesity problems among black women deserves exploration.

The role that social context—families, peer groups, neighborhoods, communities—plays in such contrasts, and generally in deterring healthy behavior and facilitating risky behavior, deserves further study. For instance, how are neighborhood factors related to racial and ethnic composition? Are neighborhood factors simply socioeconomic in origin, or are there modifiable features that could be made more favorable to healthy behavior even in the absence of reductions in poverty? Systematic data on neighborhoods could be collected (Morenoff and Lynch, 2004; Raudenbush and Sampson, 1999), and geographical analysis of national data sets could focus on "very small areas" (Bond Huie et al., 2002; see also Chandra and Skinner, 2004).

The focus of research in this area has been largely on blacks and whites, and, to a lesser extent, on Hispanics. Work is desirable to clarify behavioral differences for the other major groups—American Indians (particularly on reservations) and Asians, as well as subgroups of these groups. The behavior of these two groups appears to provide clear contrasts with whites, but the analysis necessary to determine whether these contrasts are at root socioeconomic has not been done. Does acculturation affect the behavior of these groups in the same way it affects Hispanics? If this could also be determined, one might have further clues to how the negative behavioral effects of acculturation might be arrested. Within the major racial and ethnic groups, subgroups may differ in behavior risk factors, which is worth attending to for the clues it might provide about the reasons for and the consequences of behavioral variation.

None of the group contrasts should be assumed to be static. Socio-economic change and acculturation modify behavior over time. Trends in behavior risk factors for racial and ethnic groups require continued monitoring. The trends are not all benign, and the reasons for them are certainly not well understood.

6

Social and Personal Resources

The social and psychological resources an individual can draw on can modify behavior risk factors or even reduce the health disadvantages of low socioeconomic status. Substantial evidence that such resources reduce the risk of various morbidity and mortality outcomes has accumulated over the past 25 years (Seeman, 1996; Seeman and Crimmins, 2001). The influence of these factors does not diminish at older ages: as Mendes de Leon and Glass (2004) document, such social factors as greater social integration and social engagement, as well as such psychological characteristics as beliefs regarding one's personal mastery and efficacy, continue to be important in old age.

SOCIAL RESOURCES

The evidence about social resources is largely observational, though studies have been replicated, have involved careful controls for the potentially confounding influence of sociodemographic, health, and life-style factors, and have used longitudinal data, with resources assessed in advance of health outcomes. As in other areas of study, however, selection factors cannot be entirely excluded. Longitudinal studies have shown that greater social integration is associated with lower risk of mortality in both middle age and old age (Mendes de Leon and Glass, 2004; Seeman et al., 1987, 1993) and of physical and cognitive impairment among older adults (Bassuk et al., 1999; Fratiglioni et al., 2000; Mendes de Leon et al., 1999, 2001; Strawbridge et al., 1996). Similar effects of social engagement—generally measured in terms of social activities with others—have been shown in other studies (Fabrigoule et al., 1995; Glass et al., 1999; Kiely et al., 2000). Greater social integration and more emotional support from others predict lower mortality after myocardial infarction (Berkman et al., 1992; Case et al., 1992; Williams et al., 1992). These factors also lead to lower mortality or better functional recovery after a stroke (Colantonio et al., 1993; Glass et al., 1993). More recently, higher levels of emotional support have been shown to protect against cognitive decline in the MacArthur Successful Aging Cohort (Seeman et al., 2001).

The importance of social engagement is also demonstrated in studies of the effect of religious involvement, which tends to increase with age. Compared with the younger population, older persons generally express a higher degree of religiosity (Greeley, 1989). Fellow church members provide emotional and material support, as well as information, advice, and spiritual benefits (Taylor and Chatters, 1988). Religious beliefs, it is argued, are an important source of hope and comfort and provide systems of meaning to help cope with stress, disability, the loss of loved ones, and the fear of impending death (Koenig et al., 1998).

A significant factor in religion is church attendance, which appears to be related to lower mortality and disability. Net of other demographic and socioeconomic factors, adults who attend church more than once a week have a one-third lower risk of death (in 8-year follow-up data of a nationally representative sample) than adults who never attend church (Hummer et al., 1999). An effect of similar magnitude has been verified for an older population (Koenig et al., 1999). Other cohort data also show that church attendance is associated with a lower risk of disability over a 12-year follow-up period, independently of the effects of a comprehensive set of other predictors of disability (Idler and Kasl, 1997). In contrast with the effects of church attendance, private religious activity and personal religiosity are not associated with better survival or reduced disability (Hummer et al., 1999; Idler and Kasl, 1997; Mendes de Leon and Glass, 2004).

Evidence regarding how social engagement affects health risks is beginning to emerge. Both community studies and laboratory work show that social relationships, particularly supportive ones, are associated with lower risk biological profiles. Community studies point to lower blood pressure, serum cholesterol, and levels of stress hormones (e.g., norepinephrine, epinephrine, cortisol) among people who report greater social integration or support than others (Seeman and McEwen, 1996; Seeman et al., 2002). Attendance at religious services, for instance, is associated with lower systolic and diastolic blood pressure among both black and white elderly people (Koenig et al., 1998). Laboratory-based experiments demonstrate that the presence of supportive others reduces cardiovascular and neuroendocrine reactivity among those exposed to challenging tasks (Seeman and

McEwen, 1996; Uchino et al., 1996). Importantly, studies also indicate negative health effects from social ties when those ties are a source of conflict and criticism (Kiecolt-Glaser, 1999; Kiecolt-Glaser et al., 1994; Seeman and McEwen, 1996).

The limited intervention research to date that attempts to enhance social networks and social support (Glass, 2000) has been disappointing, though this may demonstrate only how complex social relationships are and how difficult it is to alter them. A few studies have targeted patient populations—those recovering from myocardial infarction (Berkman et al., 2003) or stroke (Glass et al., 2000)—or caregivers for those with chronic conditions, such as Alzheimer's (Pillemer et al., 2000). These studies have shown little evidence of positive effects on subsequent health outcomes, possibly because of the severity of the health problems involved.

The recently completed Enhancing Recovery in Coronary Heart Disease (ENRICHD) trial (a major intervention study designed to assist socially isolated or depressed myocardial infarction patients) exemplifies the difficulties inherent in intervention efforts. The intervention, designed to build social skills and reduce depression, could not be fully implemented. Because of logistical and scheduling problems, participants randomized to the intervention had fewer than half the planned "social/cognitive intervention" sessions, and less than one-third of them actually received group therapy in addition to the initial individual therapy (Powell, 2002). The inability to provide all the group therapy intended may have substantially weakened the trial; preliminary evidence indicates that those who did have a group experience had a lower recurrence rate of fatal or nonfatal myocardial infarction than those who did not, after adjusting for important confounder variables (Saab, 2002).

Intervention efforts such as ENRICHD have largely focused on individual patients or their families, leaving untouched their larger social worlds. As has been shown for other efforts at behavior change, the broad environment constrains people's ability to maintain behavior change over time (Syme, 2002). Modifying an environment and changing social institutions is of course a substantial task, but for institutions that already play an important role in maintaining health, some interventions may be productive. In recent years, some religious institutions have become important sites for health screening and health interventions. Church-based interventions have increased fruit and vegetable consumption (Resnicow et al., 2001); increased weight loss (McNabb et al., 1997; Oexmann et al., 2001); lowered blood pressure (Oexmann et al., 2001); reduced energy intake, dietary fat, and sodium intake (Yanek et al., 2001); and increased screening for breast, cervical, colon, and prostate cancer (Erwin et al., 1999; Mann et al., 2000). It is not known whether they are more effective at this than other community organizations.

PERSONAL RESOURCES

Personal psychological characteristics are also related to health risks. Personal mastery beliefs, beliefs that one has the ability to control outcomes, have been shown to predict lower mortality in both U.S. and European populations (Bobak et al., 1998; Dalgard and Lund Haheim, 1998; Seeman and Lewis, 1997). Given that most adults spend a large portion of their time in a work setting, it is not surprising that aspects of control with respect to one's job are particularly consequential with respect to risks for cardiovascular disease (Bosma et al., 1997; Marmot et al., 1997a; Siegrist et al., 1990), as well as mortality (Amick et al., 2002; Theorell et al., 1998). The biological plausibility of a link between perceptions of control and health is suggested by a number of experimental studies showing that exposure to situations characterized by lower control is associated with enhanced physiological stress reactivity (Bohlin et al., 1986a, 1986b; Breier et al., 1987; Frankenhaeuser and Johansson, 1986).

Interventions designed to enhance perceptions of control in both work environments and nursing homes provide suggestive evidence that enhancing control can reduce health risks. Several studies in Sweden have suggested that interventions within the work environment can lower cardiovascular risk profiles (Orth-Gomer et al., 1994; Theorell et al., 2001). In nursing home studies, Langer and Rodin (1976; Rodin and Langer, 1977) demonstrated increased activity and well-being and reduced mortality among residents who are given greater opportunities to control their environment.

Self-efficacy beliefs represent a similar construct to control beliefs, focusing on the perception of one's ability to successfully perform various activities. Stronger self-efficacy characterizes individuals who believe they have more power to affect events and alter outcomes in their lives. Individuals with weaker self-efficacy beliefs are at significantly greater risk, at older ages, of cognitive (Albert et al., 1995; Seeman et al., 1996) and physical impairments (Mendes de Leon et al., 1996; Seeman et al., 1999). One possible reason for this finding is that older adults with stronger self-efficacy beliefs are more likely to exercise regularly (McAuley, 1993). Such exercise has potentially far-reaching health effects because regular physical activity reduces risks for many health outcomes, including heart disease and physical and cognitive impairment, as well as overall mortality. Interventions to encourage adoption and persistence of regular exercise of some type—especially needed given that 40 percent or fewer older adults report regular physical activity (Darnay, 1994)—may need to consider whether self-efficacy beliefs can be reinforced.

RACIAL AND ETHNIC VARIATION

Despite the evidence of effects of social and personal resources on health, the contribution of these effects to racial and ethnic health differences has received little systematic study. Some studies of religious involvement do suggest that its effects can be different between groups. Steffen et al. (2001) found that attempts to cope through religion (through prayer, trusting in God and seeking God's help, and finding comfort in religion) were related to lower blood pressure during normal daily activities and during sleep for blacks but not whites. And Musick et al. (1998) determined that religious activity was linked to fewer depressive symptoms among elderly blacks with cancer but not among whites.

Culture may in some cases lead to psychological dispositions having opposite effects among different groups. A few studies suggest that, for Korean Americans in contrast with whites, a perceived external locus of control rather than higher self-efficacy is more effective at relieving psychological distress (Bjorck et al., 1997; Kim, 2002; Sastry and Ross, 1998). Whether other social and personal resources also have different implications for the health of different groups is difficult to say. And what such studies add up to—what health differences might be accounted for—has not been investigated.

The lack of research on group differences is somewhat surprising in light of occasional suggestions that such factors may explain racial and ethnic differences. For instance, a lack of social and psychological resources in poor communities may be postulated to contribute to poorer health outcomes, or, in the case of Hispanics and Asians, social cohesiveness may be postulated to lead to unexpectedly good health outcomes. Nevertheless, the vast majority of research to date on health effects of social and psychological factors does not focus on ethnicity, treating it instead as a covariate to be controlled in multivariate models. As outlined by Mendes de Leon and Glass (2004), available evidence does not point to large or systematic differences in social resources by race or ethnicity. An important caveat here is that the evidence largely involves comparisons of whites and blacks, with only minimal information on Hispanics and little or no information about other growing ethnic populations, such as Asian subgroups.

NEEDED RESEARCH

While evidence accumulates that social and psychological resources affect health in old age, their contribution to racial and ethnic differences remains largely unstudied. Though it is plausible to postulate that such resources contribute to health differences, evidence is essential for understanding and designing possible interventions.

Research Need 9: Characterize the distribution of social and psychological resources in different older populations and investigate whether their effects on health vary by race and ethnicity.

Research on such resources, particularly for groups other than whites and blacks, is presently quite limited, leaving it unclear whether or not there are important differences that could have consequences for health. Even in the unlikely circumstance that patterns of social support, religious involvement, and psychological coping styles are found to be similar across groups, it is still plausible that they would have different implications for promoting healthy behavior, deterring risky behavior, facilitating care, and ultimately improving health.

Social and psychological factors are not identical, though they are probably interdependent. Such factors as social support and the social environment of individuals may condition the health effects of psychological coping styles, and vice versa. The degree of interdependence may vary across ethnic groups.

Research should attend to the role of these processes over the life course. Social environments and coping styles evolve and adjust as people age, being modified by and modifying individual choices. For instance, one's social network shrinks in old age, tending to focus increasingly on those who can satisfy emotional and physical needs (Mendes de Leon and Glass, 2004). The consequences of this change for health, and particularly how such dynamics play out for different racial and ethnic groups, is poorly charted.

7

Prejudice and Discrimination

Studies of race and health frequently invoke racism, prejudice, and discrimination as possible reasons for high levels of morbidity and mortality among black (Jackson et al., 1996; Krieger, 1999; Williams and Neighbors, 2001) and among other racial and ethnic minorities (e.g., Amaro et al., 1987; Salgado de Snyder, 1987). Definitions of these terms vary, and no definitions are universally accepted (Clark, 2004). For our purposes, we use these terms somewhat interchangeably as indicating negative attitudes toward or biased treatment of one group by another (Williams et al., 2003).

Various types of racism have been described (Jones, 1997): personal, which may be considered the same as prejudice (Allport, 1958); institutional, involving a set of environmental conditions, such as housing market conditions, that favors one group over another; and cultural, referring to shared beliefs about the superiority of one group over another. Racism also often involves control by one group over resources that another group wants or needs (Jones, 1997).

Discrimination refers to unequal treatment based on group membership. What actual perceptions, attitudes, or behaviors these constructs refer to depends on the context—the nature and timing of events, their frequency, severity, and duration, whether they are acute or chronic—and on how they are perceived and interpreted, whether intent is attributed, and how they may later be distorted in memory (Williams et al., 2003).

Prejudice, discrimination, and racism could affect health in several ways. First, discrimination could determine a group's living conditions and life chances, affecting such areas as education, employment, and housing.

As we note above, low socioeconomic status is one of the most important predictors of adverse changes in health status (Anderson and Armstead, 1995; Williams, 1990; Williams and Collins, 1995), though the specific mechanisms by which low status compromises health have yet to be adequately elucidated (Anderson and Armstead, 1995; Clark et al., 1999). Similarly, all the mechanisms by which discrimination limits economic and social opportunities still need to be fully accounted for (Williams and Collins, 2001), but that it has historically had an effect on minority socioeconomic status is unquestioned.

Second, discrimination could lead to differences in access to and quality of health care (Blendon et al., 1989; Council on Ethical and Judicial Affairs, 1990; Institute of Medicine, 2002), a possibility we examine in Chapter 10. Third, the experience of specific incidents of unfair treatment on the basis of race or ethnicity may generate psychic distress and other changes in physiological processes that adversely affect health (Clark, 2004; Clark et al., 1999; Landrine and Klonoff, 1996; McNeilly et al., 1996). Fourth, some of the coping strategies that people use as they grapple with inequitable living conditions and a hostile psychosocial environment, such as internalizing negative stereotypes (White et al., 2000) or using drugs and alcohol (Jackson and Ramon, 2002), may also impair physical and psychological functioning (Clark, 2004).

We focus in the rest of this chapter on the third effect, with some reference to the fourth.

Early literature on black health, especially mental health, reflects a clear consensus that racism and discrimination have adverse effects (e.g., McCarthy and Yancey, 1971). That some degree of discrimination continues is clear: for example, audit studies continue to document discrimination in housing and employment (Fix and Struyk, 1993). However, there have been comparatively few attempts to explore empirically the health effects of such discrimination among blacks, whether on children, adolescents, or adults (Jackson et al., 1996; Landrine and Klonoff, 1996; Thompson, 1996; Utsey and Ponterotto, 1996). There have been even fewer empirical studies of any kind on other racial and ethnic groups (Williams et al., 2003). Researchers have continued to note that discrimination is an important factor in understanding black health status, and some suggest that it may account for particular patterns of association (Landrine and Klonoff, 1996). Fernando (1984) even proposed that racial discrimination does not just add to stress; it is an actual pathogen. Nevertheless, these constructs and arguments have received limited empirical attention (Harrell et al., 1998; Krieger, 1999), especially as they relate to the life course and aging.

The evidence that the experience of discrimination affects health outcomes is therefore spotty. The majority of reports that have looked at this issue do document an association between the experience of unequal treatment and a variety of health outcomes, including psychological distress, blood pressure, and mental health functioning (Harrell et al., 2003). But prospective studies of the long-term effects of chronic discrimination have not been conducted.

CORRELATIONAL STUDIES

A recent review (Williams et al., 2003) identifies 53 separate community-based epidemiological studies of the association of experiences and perceptions of discrimination with health outcomes. Most of the U.S. studies have involved blacks, but there are some studies of other minorities, and studies have been conducted with immigrant groups in such other countries as Canada, England, and the Netherlands. The majority of the studies find that the self-reported experience of discrimination has an unfavorable effect, producing psychological distress, reduced psychological well-being, lowered self-esteem, impaired mental health, and even definable psychiatric disorders.

These correlational studies have also commonly examined self-reported overall health. More than 70 percent of the studies report poorer health among those who report discrimination. The studies have shown somewhat more variable relationships of discrimination to more specific health indicators. Blood pressure, an important health status measure, has sometimes been positively associated with discrimination, but sometimes has had no association or even a negative association. Cigarette smoking and alcohol use have also been linked to discrimination. Some studies attempt to show that perceptions of discrimination, net of socioeconomic factors, account for racially related health differences.

Systematic investigation of the role of discrimination in health over the life course is rare (Williams and Neighbors, 2001). One longitudinal panel study did find that reports of discrimination that were related to poorer health in the first year were still linked, 13 years later, to poorer mental health, though by that time they were related, somewhat surprisingly, to better self-reported physical health (Jackson et al., 1996). Another study that used reports of the experience of chronic discrimination found that these were related to subclinical carotid artery disease for black but not white premenopausal women (Troxel et al., 2003).

EXPERIMENTAL AND PHYSIOLOGICAL STUDIES

Harrell et al. (2003) recently reviewed 13 experimental studies of discrimination and health. Some studies focused on using analogs to racially charged stimuli in the laboratory and examining physiological reactions. For the most part, these studies show that such stimuli increase physiological arousal. What is unclear is how this response differs from arousal due to other stressors, such as those that would provoke anger.

A second set of studies tested the significance of past sensitization to racist stressors, with individuals who previously experienced discrimination assigned to various experimental conditions. Harrell et al. (2003) report, for instance, that individuals who embrace basic American values tend to be more reactive to racist material than other people.

Finally, a series of studies investigated whether physiological response is moderated by cultural affinities or personality factors, such as "John Henryism," a dispositional orientation that leads individuals to work hard in the face of impossible barriers (James et al., 1984). These studies have shown mixed results. Harrell et al. (2003) argue that they show the need for more and better studies of basic physiological processes, particularly on cholinergic pathways that link anxiety and stress to cardiovascular reactions. To explain these linkages, the authors propose new models of allostasis and allodynamism that define physiological set points and the mechanisms that govern them. The argument is that both external stressors, such as the experience of discrimination, and internal processes alter these physiological set points, which has health implications. Harrell et al. (2003) suggest that studies in this area might use pharmacological blocks and brain imaging.

NEEDED RESEARCH

These correlational and experimental studies suggest that the subjective experience of bias and unequal treatment could affect particular health outcomes. However, the evidence is uneven and inconclusive, as almost every individual study has substantial inadequacies. Across the variety of studies, the definition and measurement of the factors of prejudice, racism, discrimination, and resulting unequal treatment are still relatively crude. Another problem is uncertain delineation of physiological pathways that serve as conduits for the effects of such factors on health. In addition, the conduits undoubtedly are affected by a host of contextual factors, such as socioeconomic status, individual host resistance factors, and coping styles and responses, as well as varying by age and possibly period and cohort.

Research into the effects of prejudice and discrimination on health differences requires some systematization. Such constructs as prejudice, discrimination, and racism have shifting definitions across studies and are often poorly operationalized. The confusion from continual redefinition makes it difficult for studies to build on one another. Measurement is also a problem, particularly the determination of discrimination from self-reports, which is the usual practice in nonexperimental studies. Response biases are possible in such data and may not be independent of response biases in self-reported health status (Williams et al., 2003). Biases could even affect longitudinal studies, when prior experiences are reinterpreted in the light of subsequent events, though some closed-cohort longitudinal studies suggest this is not a critical issue (Jackson et al., 1996).

Methodological problems go beyond measurement, however, and require better study design (Krieger, 1999; Williams et al., 2003). Longitudinal studies are clearly superior to correlational studies (and avoid the methodological and ethical issues involved in discriminatory treatment of experimental subjects), but they also have limitations, which they generally share with other studies of the effects of stress. Selection processes, memory distortions, and period events with broad effects on cohorts can all complicate the design and interpretation of results. Dealing with all such issues in an efficient design would be the goal, but it is not easy to achieve.

Research Need 10: Determine the lifetime effects of prejudice and discrimination on health using longitudinal data and a framework that centers on stress and its effects.

Stressful events and experiences have been reliably linked to heath outcomes, as we discuss in the next chapter. However, what roots stress may have in prejudice and discrimination (Myers and Hwang, 2004; Pearlin, 1989) require better delineation. There is a need to distinguish among traumatic events and between macro- and microstressors (Williams et al., 2003), and the relationships may be complicated. Discriminatory experiences may combine with other life stressors that affect health. But stress resulting from discrimination may be less easy to deal with through normal coping responses than stress from other sources, and different groups may have generally different ways of dealing with stress. For instance, active and passive coping responses work as well for blacks in response to normal life stressors (low income, negative life events, deaths of relatives and friends, etc.) as for other groups, but blacks are reported to have relatively few effective coping responses to poor treatment due to racial prejudice (Jackson et al., 2003).

The effects of discrimination on the experience of stress and health outcomes may involve lags and host resistance factors and may change over the life course, influenced by personality and other life experiences, such as resource acquisition, exposure, and support processes. Effects related to aging have to be seen in the context of period and cohort variation. Experiences of discrimination may be tied to particular periods or significant historical events (such as the 1960s civil rights movement). And birth cohorts each have their own history, possibly reacting to events differently because of the stage in the life course at which the events are experienced. A framework that combines aging, period, and cohort factors is therefore needed to understand how early experiences may lead to a cascade of subsequent health-relevant events and how experiences may have different effects over the life course. Such a framework is also needed to put scientific observations in context, since these observations necessarily pertain to particular periods and may be of limited relevance to individuals late in the life course. Models for the complex biopsychosocial processes involved in stress reactions to the experience of discrimination also require development (Clark et al., 1999; Harrell et al., 2003; Williams et al., 2003), as we discuss further in the next chapter.

Research Need 11: Evaluate the effects of prejudice and discrimination on the health of minorities other than blacks.

Other racial and ethnic groups, such as American Indians and Alaska Natives, have been subject to prejudice over long periods. Immigrants have also been discriminated against, though as they assimilate and new immigrants enter, the targets shift. Arab Americans and Muslims are the latest to feel targeted. Yet indicators for the health of older adults in these groups are more favorable than indicators for blacks—and indicators actually deteriorate for immigrants as they assimilate and prejudice presumably declines. Does prejudice have effects on health in these groups, but are the effects counterbalanced by other factors, such as immigrant selectivity or better socioeconomic status? Or is prejudice against these groups weaker or less pervasive, of a different quality, or for some reason less consequential for health than among blacks? The answers could have implications not only for these racial and ethnic groups, but also for understanding the mechanisms that link prejudice and health for any group.

8

Stress

One frequently mentioned explanation for racial and ethnic health differences is the role of stress. The general hypothesis is that greater exposure to stress over the life course increases susceptibility to morbidity and mortality among members of minority groups. This hypothesis rests on three assumptions: (1) that stress itself is related to illness and longevity; (2) that, compared to whites, members of the minority groups at risk experience higher levels of stress, either at given points or cumulatively over time; and (3) that greater exposure to stress accounts for a substantial portion of the health disadvantage of the minorities at risk.

STRESS AND HEALTH

Stress may be defined as "environmental demands that tax or exceed the adaptive capacity of an organism, resulting in biological and psychological changes that may be detrimental and place the organism at risk for disease" (Cohen et al., 1998) or disability. Stressors can take many forms, including those associated with economic difficulties, physical deprivation, low status, occupational strain, death of a spouse or loved one, family responsibilities or difficulties, neighborhood instability, and discrimination. Stress is often assessed by using rating scales for stressful life events or it is determined by magnitude of exposure to specific stressors (e.g., job stress) or the presence or absence of a chronic stressor (e.g., caregiving responsibilities).

The connection between stress and morbidity and mortality has been demonstrated in a variety of studies. Stressful life events have been shown to predict mortality in initially healthy populations (Rosengren et al., 1993) and in patients with heart disease (Ruberman et al., 1984). Specific types of stressful events are also linked to mortality and illness. In particular, job strain, bereavement, and providing care for a chronically ill relative have been predictive of all-cause mortality and heart disease (Karasek et al., 1988; Martikainen and Valkonen, 1996; Schnall et al., 1994; Schulz and Beach, 1999).

One type of stressor—caring for a spouse with Alzheimer's disease—is especially relevant for older adults. Although caregiving can have some emotional rewards, caregivers on the whole report extraordinarily high levels of burden and stress (Schulz et al., 1995; Vitaliano et al., 1997), which may increase their mortality risk. A recent study compared 392 older people who were providing care for a spouse with a group of 400 people of the same age without this responsibility. Approximately 50 percent of the caregivers reported emotional strain associated with their caregiver roles. Over the 4-year study, those caregivers who reported mental and emotional strain were 63 percent more likely to die than the noncaregivers. Caregivers not reporting strain were not at increased risk of mortality (Schulz and Beach, 1999). There is therefore at least moderately strong evidence that stress is predictive of morbidity and mortality.

The association between stress and illness may be indirect, in that stress has been shown to influence a number of other risk factors. Stress has been associated with an increase in intravenous drug use, smoking, alcohol use, physical inactivity, and unprotected sex (Dougal and Baum, 2001; Kaplan et al., 1993). Therefore, stress may be looked at as both a potential proximal and distal cause of illness and mortality.

RACE, ETHNICITY, AND STRESS

The Commonwealth Minority Health Survey provides a unique glimpse of racial and ethnic variation in stress (Williams, 2000). On a global measure combining exposure to stressors in five domains (occupation, finances, relationships, racial bias, and violence), blacks, Hispanics, and Asians reported higher levels of stress than whites. Among Hispanics, Puerto Ricans had the highest levels of stress. Interestingly, there was dramatic variation among the Asian subgroups included: Chinese reported higher levels of stress than any other group in the study, Vietnamese were intermediate, and Koreans reported the lowest levels in the study.

Reaction to stressors may also differ across groups. Blacks, especially those at the low end of the economic spectrum, report not only a great number of stressful life events but also stronger responses to them, or greater distress, than whites in a variety of domains (Myers and Hwang, 2004). In some studies, though not all, minorities, especially blacks, react with greater psychological distress than whites to unpleasant events (Mirowsky and Ross, 1990; Myers et al., 2002; Ulbrich et al., 1989; Warheit et al., 1973).

Differences in exposure to stress are partly attributable to group differences in socioeconomic status (Neff, 1984; Warheit et al., 1975). However, race may also interact with socioeconomic status in producing levels of distress. Kessler and Neighbors (1986) found such a race-by-class interaction, such that low-status blacks reported higher levels of distress than high-status blacks or whites of any status. In contrast, after controlling for status, older blacks in the recent Macarthur Study of Successful Aging reported *lower* levels of distress than older whites. In particular, low-status blacks had lower levels of distress than low-status whites (Kubzansky et al., 2000). Thus, although race and socioeconomic status appear to interact in affecting stress responses, the direction of this interaction is far from clear. In addition, exposure to and the experience of stress for some minority groups may be lower than for whites. In one study (Uppaluri et al., 2001), for instance, Asian Indians and Koreans reported lower levels of stress response over a 2-week period than whites, and immigrants who had lived in the United States less than 1 year reported significantly lower stress response levels than those who had lived in the United States for at least 15 years.

Some stressors may decline in importance for older people; others may become more significant. Retrospective reports of discrimination decline with age. Nevertheless, for current generations of minority older adults, stress due to racism and discrimination may be especially important, given that their life histories extend back to earlier periods when civil rights received less attention. Minority older adults may also have greater exposure than younger cohorts to potential stressors related to acculturative stress, spousal and family caregiving, and raising grandchildren (which can of course also be emotionally rewarding; Myers and Hwang, 2004). However, it is unclear, with regard to family responsibilities, whether minority older adults feel as burdened as their white counterparts. Black and Hispanic grandparents care for grandchildren more often than whites do, but the subjective burden they experience may be less (Myers and Hwang, 2004).

In addition to stress, there may be other psychological factors that are predictive of health outcomes and important for racial and ethnic health differences. For instance, depression, anxiety, and anger or hostility have all been prospectively linked with increased cardiovascular or all-cause mortality (Rozanski et al., 1999). Interestingly, each of these psychological factors is believed to be triggered by stressful life experiences. Few if any studies have examined whether these psychological factors contribute to health differences.

NEEDED RESEARCH

Does greater experience of and exposure to chronic stress account for some racial and ethnic health differences among older adults? This question has yet to be systematically investigated; the evidence is incomplete and so far inconclusive. Better measurement of relevant dimensions of stress would be critical to understanding whether and how it affects health differences. While rating scales try to encompass the variety of sources, how adequately they do so is unclear. Such dimensions of the stressful experience as exposure, appraisal, and response (Lobel et al., 1992) require attention.

Research Need 12: Study populations of different racial and ethnic groups to assess the connection between health and the stresses that accumulate over a lifetime.

Despite the considerable research on stress and health, it is still unclear what role stress plays in the health of older adults of different groups. Some minorities, especially blacks and Hispanics, appear to experience higher levels of chronic stress, but it has not been determined whether this is linked to relatively higher morbidity and mortality as they age. Various stressors may be of concern for different groups—discrimination and racism, as discussed above, but also socioeconomic pressure, acculturative stress for immigrant populations, the stress of family responsibilities, and aging-related problems. Research should focus on sources of stress that apply particularly to minority populations and on the suggestions in the literature that reactions to stressful events may vary across groups.

The assessment of cumulative stresses over the life course should be given special attention and may be especially relevant. People who have experienced more "lifetime adversities" have been shown to exhibit potentially pathogenic physiological activity (Singer and Ryff, 1999). Older minorities, especially blacks and perhaps other groups, have complex life histories that often involve substantial adversity. Investigation of how this affects health in old age, with attention to cohort and historical effects, is a fruitful direction for investigation.

Several psychological factors are associated with stress, including depression, anxiety, and anger or hostility, and may also play a role in health differences. Although a good deal of research has examined the effects of these factors on morbidity and mortality, little of this research has focused exclusively on older adults, and even less has focused on racial and ethnic differences.

9

Biopsychosocial Interactions

The factors we have considered so far—including selectivity, socio-economic status, health behaviors, prejudice and discrimination, social support, and stress—are typically studied independently, often within the boundaries of separate disciplines. Yet a good deal of research indicates that these factors do not affect health independently but interact among themselves and with biological systems. The study of psychosocial and biological interactions, referred to as biopsychosocial or biobehavioral research, has demonstrated profound effects on biological systems of an array of factors. For instance, psychosocial and behavioral factors have been shown to affect organ systems (e.g., the cardiovascular, neuroendocrine, central nervous, and immune systems) and cellular (e.g., synaptic connections) and molecular (e.g., RNA) factors (Anderson, 1998).

Examination of links to the biological level is critical to understanding health differences in late life because the biological level serves as the pathway to disease and death. A number of studies have found significant racial and ethnic group differences in several biological measures, including the well-known differences in blood pressure, low-density and high-density cholesterol, and obesity, and, more recently, in response to pharmacological agents (Burroughs et al., 2002; James, 1999; Kumanyika, 1987; Whiteley et al., 1999; Zoratti, 1998). Biological factors should not be studied in isolation but as part of a system in which psychosocial, behavioral, and environmental factors lead to potentially pathogenic changes, in ways that may vary by racial or ethnic group.

Researchers in this area have identified candidate biological markers or mechanisms that may be related to psychosocial, behavioral, and environmental factors and may also be associated with risk for disease. These mechanisms include physiological reactivity, allostatic load, psychoneuroimmunology, metabolic syndrome, and neurovisceral integration.

PHYSIOLOGICAL REACTIVITY

Physiological reactivity is defined as the magnitude of changes in some physiological system in response to acute psychological or behavioral stress. The changes most often studied, typically under laboratory conditions, involve cardiovascular reactivity (e.g., heart rate, blood pressure). The hypothesis is that frequently activated and exaggerated cardiovascular responses to stress raise resting blood pressure levels over time and damage coronary arteries (Matthews et al., 1986; Turner et al., 1992). The strongest evidence for this hypothesis comes from animal experiments that demonstrate an etiological role for stress-induced reactivity in both coronary heart disease (Manuck et al., 1990, 1995) and hypertension (Hallback, 1975; Lovallo and Wilson, 1992; Manuck et al., 1990). Among humans there is evidence that individuals at risk for hypertension—due to a family history or older age, being black or having borderline hypertension—may also exhibit cardiovascular hyperreactivity to stress (Turner et al., 1992). There is also emerging evidence in humans that cardiovascular reactivity among healthy individuals may be prospectively related to later hypertension (Carroll et al., 2001; Falkner et al., 1981; Light et al., 1992; Menkes et al., 1989). Finally, research is emerging on a possible negative correlation between socioeconomic status and reactivity (Gump et al., 1999).

In a new line of research on reactivity, acute psychological stress has been shown to elicit myocardial ischemia, an imbalance between the blood supply to the heart and the demands placed on it to supply the body with oxygenated blood. Myocardial ischemia may result in angina pain, but it is frequently silent, occurring without pain. Psychological stress has been shown to produce silent ischemia in the laboratory; such responses are predictive of ischemia in real life, as measured by ambulatory cardiac recording (Blumenthal et al., 1995). In patients with a history of heart disease, ischemia induced by psychological stress is prospectively related to subsequent cardiac events (Jiang et al., 1996).

A number of studies have explored differences between blacks and whites in stress-induced reactivity as a possible reason for group differences in hypertension. These studies generally find a tendency among black adults and children toward greater peripheral vascular responses to stress in comparison with whites (Anderson, 1989). Blacks show greater cardiovascular responses in laboratory research to stimuli associated with racism (e.g., films depicting racist incidents, imagery related to racism) than to nonracist stimuli (Armstead et al., 1989; Guyll et al., 2001). Blacks also show greater blood pressure reactivity than whites to discrimination and unfair treatment (Guyll et al., 2001). However, the contribution of such responses to black-white differences in the prevalence of hypertension has not been determined.

ALLOSTATIC LOAD

Allostatic load is another concept developed to explain how psychosocial factors might affect biological systems in potentially pathogenic ways (McEwen and Stellar, 1993). It is defined as the overtaxing of several physiological systems ("wear and tear") in response to stress or other psychosocial or behavioral factors, so that dysregulation and possibly disease may develop. The concept of allostatic load incorporates the notion of physiological reactivity, but it also includes other physiological changes that might be pathogenic. Those changes include having a chronically high level of resting physiological activity (e.g., high levels of stress hormones or high blood pressure); an exaggerated physiological response to psychosocial challenges; the relative inability of the physiological system to recover after acute stress; and, over time, an inadequate physiological response to stress (low reactivity) due to fatigue or dysfunction, which triggers potentially harmful compensatory responses from other systems (McEwen, 1998; Myers and Hwang, 2004). In essence, allostatic load represents a cumulative, multisystems perspective on physiological risk.

Recent research on the Macarthur Successful Aging Cohort indicates that high levels of allostatic load predict morbidity and mortality among older adults. For instance, Seeman et al. (1997) have discovered that higher allostatic load scores are prospectively associated with increased incidence of cardiovascular disease and increased risk for decline in cognitive and physical functioning in older adults. Allostatic load scores have been found to be higher among persons with lower educational attainment and higher levels of hostility than average, suggesting a potential role for allostatic load in the greater disease risk in these populations (Kubzansky et al., 1999). To date, racial and ethnic group differences in allostatic load and the role of such differences in health differences have not been explored.

PSYCHONEUROIMMUNOLOGY

Psychoneuroimmunology is defined as the examination of the interactions among psychological, behavioral, and social factors with immunological and neuroendocrine outcomes. It is now well established that psychological factors, especially chronic stress, can lead to impairments in immune system functioning in both the young and older adults (Kiecolt-Glaser and Glaser, 1995). In several studies of older adults, those who are providing care for a relative with dementia report high levels of stress and exhibit significant impairments in immune system functioning when compared with non-caregivers (Kiecolt-Glaser et al., 1987). Stress-induced changes in the immune system may affect a number of outcomes, including slowing the wound healing process and increasing susceptibility to infections (Cohen and Williamson, 1991; Cohen et al., 1991; Kiecolt-Glaser et al., 1995).

To date, there have been few if any published studies on racial and ethnic group differences in stress-induced immunosuppression and into the role it may play in health differences.

THE METABOLIC SYNDROME AND PSYCHOSOCIAL FACTORS

The metabolic syndrome, also known as syndrome X or the insulin resistance syndrome, is characterized by a combination of central adiposity (abdominal fat), insulin resistance, glucose intolerance, and hypertension (Reaven, 1988). The metabolic syndrome has been prospectively linked to type 2 diabetes and cardiovascular disease prevalence and mortality (Baillie et al., 1998; Laaksonen et al., 2002; Lakka et al., 2002; Vague and Raccah, 1992).

Research has uncovered some racial and ethnic differences in metabolic syndrome and its components. In particular, blacks exhibit higher levels of central obesity, insulin resistance, hypertension, and glucose intolerance than whites (Adams-Campbell et al., 1990; Kasim-Karakas, 2000; Lovejoy et al., 1996). Research on the relationship of psychosocial factors and metabolic syndrome is emerging, and there is some evidence of a significant link. For example, Brunner and associates have found an inverse relationship between socioeconomic status and metabolic syndrome, a connection that might be mediated by heightened sympathetic nervous system activity (Brunner et al., 1997, 2002; see also Hjemdahl, 2002). In a prospective analysis of older men, Vitaliano et al. (2002) found that the chronic stress of caregiving for a person with Alzheimer's was a predictor of metabolic syndrome, which in turn was discovered to mediate the connection between chronic stress and coronary heart disease. Research has not determined whether racial or ethnic differences in metabolic syndrome are mediated by stress or other psychosocial factors or the role of metabolic syndrome in different disease outcomes by group.

NEUROVISCERAL INTEGRATION

Thayer and Friedman (2004) have proposed a model of neurovisceral integration as a new framework that could possibly link research on psychosocial factors to health outcomes. The model complements and extends previous biopsychosocial models, positing a common element among them: an imbalance between the branches of the autonomic nervous system (ANS), the parasympathetic and sympathetic, that favors the latter. The status of the ANS at any time is a function of the inhibitory influences of the parasympathetic system and the excitatory effects of the sympathetic system. The ANS is important since it controls cardiovascular, neuroendocrine, and immune system functions; it also interacts with key brain regions related to psychological and emotional processes. Thayer and Friedman (2004) hypothesize that the lessening of parasympathetic influence in the ANS (as indexed by heart rate variability), especially under psychosocial challenges such as stress, worry, perseverative thinking, depression, anxiety, racism, and low status, may be a key biological pathway that underlies racial and ethnic differences in health in late life.

Although this model has not been evaluated with respect to health differences, there is evidence that lowered heart rate variability and a higher resting heart rate (as an index of decreased parasympathetic tone) are related to increased all-cause mortality (Thayer and Friedman, 2004).

These biobehavioral models of disease should not be viewed as competing conceptualizations, since there is considerable overlap among them. Cardiovascular reactivity, allostatic load, immune system changes, metabolic syndrome, and heart rate variability are strongly correlated. At this time, it is not clear which of these, or any other biobehavioral model, is most predictive of illness and death. Nevertheless, these models are likely to be related to many of the proposed determinants of health differences, such as stress, social support, racism, health risk behaviors, and socioeconomic status, and may therefore indicate mechanisms through which such risk factors translate into disease susceptibility and health differences.

NEEDED RESEARCH

Much basic research is still needed on biopsychosocial mechanisms, and further work is needed to elucidate the links, if any, with race and ethnicity.

Research Need 13: Clarify how biopsychosocial factors affect health outcomes over time in racial and ethnic groups of middle-aged and older adults.

It has been hypothesized that psychosocial effects on biopsychosocial outcomes, such as cardiovascular reactivity, allostatic load, psychoneuro-immunology, metabolic syndrome, and neurovisceral integration are predictors of morbidity and mortality. It remains an empirical question whether they indeed affect health among older adults and whether they have different implications for health across racial and ethnic groups.

Basic research is needed on all these potential disease pathways for the effects of acute and chronic stress, as well as on how these mechanisms mediate between such stressors as racism and low status and health outcomes for various racial and ethnic groups. The discovery of differences in such mechanisms, in their linkages to social factors or in their effects on health, would provide evidence of their involvement in differences. Besides longitudinal studies, laboratory experiments and ambulatory studies of physiological activity in the natural environment would be informative. For instance, exploring the biological concomitants of group differences in neighborhood environments and occupational experiences might provide a better understanding of their differential effects across groups.

10

Health Care

Racial and ethnic minorities may face challenges in having access to medical care in the United States. When they receive it, their care may not be equivalent to that for other groups. Why this is so, however, is a complex issue involving not only possible differences in ability to pay and provider behavior, but also in such factors as patient preferences, differential treatment by providers, and geographical variability.

INSURANCE COVERAGE

Blacks, Hispanics, and some Asian populations, when compared with whites, appear to have lower levels of health insurance coverage, with Hispanics facing greater barriers to health insurance than any other group (Institute of Medicine, 2002). However, Hispanics and Asians are considerably heterogeneous in insurance coverage, as Table 10-1 shows for the adult population under 65 (Collins et al., 2002; Doty and Ives, 2002; Hughes 2002). Uninsured rates are much higher for Mexicans and Central Americans than for Puerto Ricans. Among Asians, Chinese, Japanese, Filipinos, and Indians have uninsured rates that are comparable to or lower than those of whites, while Koreans and Vietnamese have higher uninsured rates than blacks.

Blacks and Hispanics are less likely to have insurance coverage from a private employer, whether directly or through a spouse, and more likely to have public health insurance coverage than whites (Blendon et al., 1989; Hogue et al., 2000; National Institutes of Health, 1998). Blacks and His-

TABLE 10-1 Health Insurance Coverage for U.S. Adults Aged 18-64, 2001

Population	Percent Uninsured	
	Currently	In Past Year
Total United States	16	24
White	12	20
Black	22	30
Hispanic	35	46
Mexican	39	49
Central American	47	55
Puerto Rican	16	35
Asian	14	21
Chinese	12	16
Korean	52	55
Vietnamese	32	37
Filipino	6	15
Indian	13	18
Japanese	1	4

SOURCES: Collins et al. (2002); Doty and Ives (2002); Hughes (2002). Data are from the Commonwealth Fund 2001 Health Care Quality Survey.

panics are also more likely than whites to receive care in nonoptimal organizational settings (such as emergency rooms) and to lack continuity in health care. Analyses of racial and ethnic differences in access to and the use of health services between 1977 and 1996 show that the black-white gap has not narrowed over time, and the gap between Hispanics and whites has widened (Weinick et al., 2000). Moreover, this study found that, even if income and health insurance coverage were equal, racial and ethnic differences in having a usual source of care and in receiving ambulatory care in the previous year would not have been eliminated, because one-half to three-quarters of the differences on these indicators were not accounted for by income and insurance coverage.

In 1965, the Medicare program was established to reduce financial barriers to hospital and physician services for persons aged 65 and older. To participate in this program, hospitals had to comply with Title VI of the Civil Rights Act of 1964, which requires that no one be excluded from federal benefits based on race, color, or national origin. This requirement played a large role in desegregating hospitals (Quadagno, 2000).

Medicare has indeed improved the situation for older adults. For instance, Decker and Rapaport (2002) show that turning 65 increases the chances of having a mammogram among black women, particularly uneducated black women. However, there is also evidence that racial differences remain among older adults in access to health services (Gornick, 2000).

TABLE 10-2 Health Care Coverage for Persons 65 Years of Age and Over, 1998 (in percent)

Insurance Type	White	Black	Hispanic
Private insurance	72.3	40.5	29.1
Private, work-based	38.8	27.6	17.8
Medicaid	5.4	18.0	27.2
Medicare only	20.9	37.9	38.4

SOURCE: Data from National Center for Health Statistics (2001).

Table 10-2 shows the level of health care coverage for black, white, and Hispanic older adults (National Center for Health Statistics, 2001). Almost all of these persons have Medicare. However, in comparison with whites, black and Hispanic older adults are considerably less likely to have private insurance and more likely to receive Medicaid or to have Medicare as their only insurance.

The limitations of Medicare create economic challenges for blacks and Hispanics. Medicare does not cover such medical needs as prescription drugs, dental care, and long-term care, and it imposes various out-of-pocket medical expenses: an annual deductible for some care, copayments on physician charges, and payment for one day of inpatient care. These expenses may represent a substantial burden for low-income older adults, and minorities are more affected because of lower household incomes. In 1996, two-thirds of white Medicare beneficiaries had incomes of less than $25,000; 90 percent of black and Hispanic beneficiaries had incomes this low (Gornick, 2000). Other data show that black and Hispanic older adults have higher rates of poverty than their white counterparts, as do Asians and American Indians and Alaska Natives (Williams and Wilson, 2001).

Many older adults reduce their out-of-pocket expenses by purchasing supplemental private insurance, but black and Hispanic older adults are a little more than twice as likely as whites not to do so (Wallace et al., 1998). Not surprisingly, although black Medicare beneficiaries report higher levels of morbidity than their white counterparts, they report lower levels of office visits and more inpatient, emergency room, and nursing home visits (Gornick, 2000). In comparison with whites, black beneficiaries also have markedly fewer visits to specialists, and they receive such diagnostic services as mammography and sigmoidoscopy much less often (Gornick, 2000). For some older persons with low incomes and limited assets, Medicaid can cover much of their out-of-pocket medical expenses. However, only about 11 percent of older Medicare beneficiaries also receive Medicaid; these dual eligibles are more likely to be in poor health and over age 85 than other Medicare beneficiaries (Feder et al., 2001).

The situation with regards to American Indians and Alaska Natives is somewhat unique because of the existence of the Indian Health Service (IHS), which operates its own network of inpatient and ambulatory care facilities. While insurance coverage is an issue—24 percent of American Indians do not have health insurance (Brown et al., 2000)—it does not factor into matters of access to care in the same manner as for other subpopulations. The tripartite system of the IHS, tribally operated clinics, and urban Indian clinics represent a unique ecology within which American Indians seek help for physical, mental, alcohol, and drug problems. This is particularly relevant when discussing health care challenges for American Indian elderly since the emphasis of the IHS system is on acute rather than chronic health problems (Baldridge, 2001). Although the IHS is intended, legally, to be a residual provider, a large fraction of the IHS-eligible population depends on it (Cunningham, 1996).

QUALITY OF CARE

Research reveals systematic racial differences in the kind and quality of medical care received by Medicare beneficiaries (Escarce et al., 1993; McBean and Gornick, 1994). In 1992, black Medicare beneficiaries were less likely than their white counterparts to receive any of the 16 most commonly performed hospital procedures (McBean and Gornick, 1994). The differences were largest for referral-sensitive procedures. The Medicare files showed only four nonelective procedures that black Medicare beneficiaries received more frequently than whites—all procedures (such as the amputation of a lower limb and the removal of both testes) that reflect delayed diagnosis or initial failure in the management of chronic disease. Since a greater percentage of black than white Medicare beneficiaries make out-of-pocket payments for deductibles and copayments (McBean and Gornick, 1994), this burden could contribute to less use of ambulatory medical care and to the postponement or avoidance of treatment.

Contrasts among different groups are evident if one focuses on a few procedures that alleviate some major sources of morbidity and mortality, procedures supported by strong scientific evidence and practitioner consensus. Jencks et al. (2000) identified 24 such measures that they labeled measures of the quality of care for Medicare beneficiaries, and 21 of these have been compared across racial and ethnic groups (Hebb et al., 2003), including such inpatient measures as warfarin for patients with atrial fibrillation and such outpatient measures as mammograms at least every 2 years. Receipt of appropriate treatment by each racial or ethnic group is compared with the percentage receiving appropriate treatment overall in Figure 10-1. Racial and ethnic minorities appear to be at some disadvantage, particularly for outpatient rather than inpatient procedures. Hispanics

96

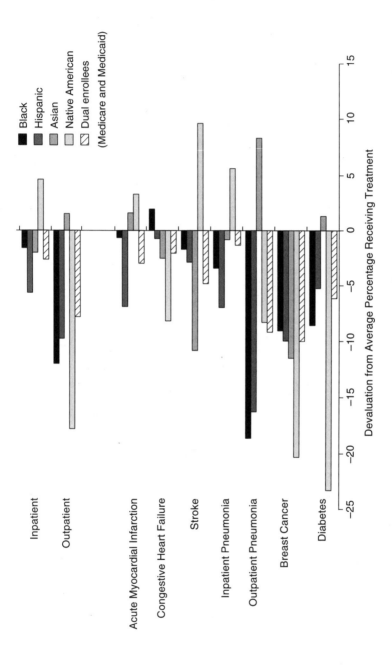

FIGURE 10-1 Treatment for minorities in comparison with all Medicare beneficiaries: Differences in percentage receiving treatment.
SOURCE: Data in Hebb et al. (2003).

and American Indians and Alaska Natives, overall, may receive care that is as inadequate as that for blacks, though because of small numbers and problems with racial and ethnic identification, the figures must be treated with caution. People enrolled in both Medicare and Medicaid (of any racial or ethnic group) also receive less adequate care than average, suggesting a socioeconomic dimension to poor care. However, their disadvantage is sometimes smaller than that of particular racial and ethnic groups.

Such differences in the receipt of medical procedures are consistent with a larger literature, generally for earlier years, that finds systematic racial and ethnic differences in the receipt of a broad spectrum of therapeutic interventions (Geiger, 2002; Institute of Medicine, 2002; Mayberry et al., 2000). Blacks and sometimes other minorities are less likely to receive a diverse range of procedures, ranging from high-technology interventions to basic diagnostic and treatment procedures, and they experience poorer quality medical care than whites.

Differences in patient preferences and inappropriate use by whites of some procedures may play a role in the differences. For instance, Schneider et al. (2001) show that the black-white difference in angioplasty can be explained by inappropriate or at least questionable use of the procedure for whites. However, they find that this explanation does not fully account for differences in bypass surgery. The pattern of differences between blacks and whites appears robust even when such factors are considered, and it persists in studies that adjust for differences in health insurance, socioeconomic status, stage and severity of disease, comorbidity, and the type of medical facility (Institute of Medicine, 2002).

Weighed against such evidence is one recent study of a nationwide sample of almost 30,000 Medicare patients hospitalized with heart failure in 1998 and 1999 (Rathore et al., 2003). Blacks were slightly more likely than whites to receive appropriate treatment (ACE inhibitors and measurement of left ventricular ejection fraction). They were more likely to be readmitted but had lower mortality rates up to a year after hospitalization. None of these differences, however, was significant after controlling for patient medical history and other patient, physician, and hospital characteristics. This study, drawing on the same database as Hebb et al. (2003) and reaching essentially similar conclusions in the area of treatment of congestive heart failure (see Figure 10-1), shows that even blacks, despite falling short of standard treatment more often than others, are not necessarily disadvantaged in every treatment area.

Some differences in quality of care may reflect the particular institutions and health care providers on which minorities depend. Regardless of insurance coverage, blacks and Hispanics are almost twice as likely as whites to receive care from a hospital-based provider (Institute of Medicine, 2002). In particular, they are almost 1.6 times more likely than whites to be treated at safety-net urban hospitals. Some evidence also suggests that minority patients are more likely than whites to be treated by less proficient physicians (Mukamel et al., 2000).

GEOGRAPHIC AND INSTITUTIONAL VARIATION

One factor that needs to be more consistently taken into account in studying racial and ethnic differences is the role of geography or residential area. Access to high-quality care varies considerably by area—by state, between rural and urban areas, as well as across smaller communities (Waidmann and Rajan, 2000; Wennberg and Cooper, 1999). Since racial and ethnic groups are unevenly distributed across communities, geographic variation in health care has the potential to explain some health care differences. For instance, states with large proportions of blacks tend to provide less appropriate treatment to all myocardial infarction patients, whether black or not, than states with smaller proportions of blacks (Chandra and Skinner, 2004).

The relationship between geographic variation and racial and ethnic differences in health care is complex. Some geographic variation may be due to racial factors related to residential segregation by race. But some variation in care is clearly not geographic, as when variations exist within geographic areas. Several studies have found racial and ethnic differences in care in a single facility (e.g., Baker et al., 1996; Chung et al., 1995; Lowe et al., 2001; Moore et al., 1994; Ng et al., 1996; Peterson et al., 1997; Todd et al., 1993, 2000); a single geographic location (Herholz et al., 1996; Ramsey et al., 1997; Segal et al., 1996); and, in the case of cardiovascular disease, even after a broad range of hospital characteristics are considered (Geiger, 2002).

Health care can also vary within health systems, though some studies show similar treatment for different racial groups. In the Veterans Administration health system, for instance (where differences in insurance coverage are minimized), black-white differences do not appear for the treatment of colorectal cancer (Dominitz et al., 1998) but have been shown in the treatment of heart disease (Oddone et al., 1998; Peterson et al., 1994; Sedlis et al., 1997; Whittle et al., 1993), gall-bladder disease (Arozullah et al., 1999), and mental health (Kales et al., 2000). In Department of Defense medical facilities, no black-white differences were found in the treatment of prostate cancer (Optenberg et al., 1995) or cervical cancer (Farley et al., 2001). Similarly, no differences were found in treatment of acute myocardial infarction through catheterization and revascularization procedures, but whites were more likely than minorities to be considered for future catheterization (Taylor et al., 1997).

To produce overall differences in care, the choice of hospitals or clinics that different groups attend and variations in treatment within those institutions could reinforce each other, or cancel each other out, or one or another factor could be more important. An example of the first possibility is one study of inadequate pain management, which found that all patients treated in settings where the patient population was primarily black or Hispanic were more likely to receive inadequate analgesia than those treated in settings where the patient population was primarily white (Cleeland et al., 1997). In addition, minority patients were more likely to be undermedicated for pain than white patients and more likely to have the severity of their pain underestimated by physicians. In contrast, in a five-state study, Kahn et al. (1994) found that blacks received poorer care in acute care hospitals than whites in the same hospitals, but because more blacks in the study were seen at higher-quality urban teaching hospitals, their overall quality of care was no worse. Finally, focusing on acute myocardial infarction, Skinner et al. (2003) found that, nationwide, blacks received care at lower-quality hospitals, where they tended to make up a larger proportion of the patients. Within groups of hospitals with different proportions of black admissions, however, white patients actually received poorer care than blacks, as reflected in 30-day mortality rates adjusted for various factors.

STEREOTYPING BY PROVIDERS

Some differences in medical care may be due to stereotypes of different groups held by health care providers. The authors of *Unequal Treatment* (Institute of Medicine, 2002) argue that unconscious or unthinking discrimination based on negative stereotypes, even in the absence of conscious prejudice, may contribute to systematic bias in care.

This argument is based on a chain of reasoning. Stereotypes are common in American society for various racial and ethnic groups. National data show that whites view blacks, Hispanics, and Asians more negatively than they view themselves, with perceptions of blacks being the most unfavorable and perceptions of Hispanics being substantially more negative than perceptions of Asians. For instance, 29 percent of whites agree with the statement that most blacks are unintelligent, while 6 percent of whites say the same of most whites. Similarly, many more whites say that most blacks are prone to violence (51 percent) than those who say the same about most whites (16 percent) (Davis and Smith, 1990; Williams, 2001b). Such stereotypes can be activated, and affect behavior, under conditions of time pressure, when quick judgments must be made on complex tasks, with cognitive overload and in the presence of such emotions as anger and anxiety (van Ryn, 2002). In the typical health care encounter, some of these conditions are present, particularly cognitive complexity and time pressure.

The possibility that some health care providers may hold particular stereotypes is suggested by a few studies in which physicians were found to view their black patients more negatively than white patients (Finucane and Carrese, 1990; van Ryn and Burke, 2000). For instance, van Ryn and Burke (2000) found that—even after adjusting for patient age, sex, socioeconomic status, sickness or frailty and overall health, and patient availability of social support—physicians viewed black patients, compared with whites, as less kind, congenial, intelligent, and educated, less likely to adhere to medical advice, and more likely to lack social support and to abuse alcohol and drugs. Experimental studies of physicians (Schulman et al., 1999; Weisse et al., 2001) and medical students (Rathore et al., 2000) provide evidence that the experimental manipulation of hypothetical patients' characteristics such as race can lead to variations in provider perceptions.

But do stereotypes actually affect patient care? There is little evidence on this issue, though one may hypothesize various possibilities. For instance, a health care provider may interpret symptoms in line with beliefs about group differences. These beliefs might be based on generalizations from clinical experience (Satel, 2000, 2001-2002), or a provider may also select treatments based on stereotypical assumptions about patient behavior. Some research tackles this latter possibility. A national sample of AIDS care physicians predicted that, among hypothetical patients, black men would be less likely to adhere to antiretroviral therapy—a generalization that may be right for some therapies but not others (see below). Since potential adherence to therapy is a factor in decisions to start treatment, the inference might be drawn that black men would be less likely to receive such care, but this potential effect of stereotypes was not actually demonstrated (Bogart et al., 2001). Somewhat similarly, van Ryn et al. (1999; cited in van Ryn and Fu, 2003) found that physicians rated black patients, in comparison with white patients, as more likely to be lacking in social support and less likely to participate in cardiac rehabilitation. The likelihood of such participation is a factor in recommending revascularization, but the researchers did not link any difference in recommendations to the stereotype.

Whether medical decisions are actually affected by stereotypes is therefore not known. It would be useful to determine how often stereotypes are activated, in what circumstances, and what medical decisions are indeed affected. In principle, stereotypes would not be a problem if treatment decisions were entirely individualized (as suggested earlier, in the genetics section, as a long-term goal). However, negative stereotypes could still make the provider-patient interaction uncomfortable, which could hamper such individualization by restricting the full exchange of information. Such processes may well be important in particular individual cases but their overall contribution to less appropriate care for minorities, or to explaining racial and ethnic differences in health in later life, remains uncertain.

PATIENT BEHAVIOR

Differences in patient self-care—a behavior about which stereotypes may exist—are themselves unconfirmed. Patient self-care covers behavior ranging from seeking health care to compliance with prescribed therapies. Compliance with complicated new therapies, such as those to control insulin-dependent diabetes and for HIV, has been shown to be better among those, including older adults, with more education. However, with education controlled, neither blacks nor Hispanics differ significantly from whites in these self-maintenance behaviors (Goldman and Smith, 2002). But other studies have documented differences by race. For instance, persistence with statin therapy among older patients—which tends to decline over time and is also related to socioeconomic status—declines more, regardless of status, among blacks and other nonwhite patients than in white patients. In fact, black subjects had 2.7 times the odds of suboptimal persistence with statin therapy compared with whites, the racial difference being greater than that on any other predictor analyzed (Benner et al., 2002).

Somewhat inconsistent results also have been shown for the use of screening tests. Winkleby and Cubbin (2004) show that, at ages 45-64, black and Hispanic women do not differ from whites with regard to having had a Pap test or a mammogram in the preceding 2 years. However, when the proportions of women having had such tests are adjusted for education and income, blacks and Hispanics are significantly more likely to be screened than whites. This result also holds for Hispanics aged 65-74; for blacks the differences were not significant at that age. However, Medicare reimbursement records tell the opposite story. Black and Hispanic women aged 52-69 less often receive a mammogram paid for under Medicare fee-for-service than the average beneficiary of this program (Figure 10-1; Hebb et al., 2003). In addition, Strzelczyk and Dignan (2002) show that non-white women in the Colorado Mammography Project are less likely than whites to adhere to a recommended follow-up screening. Such apparent inconsistencies may have explanations, but they suggest that the role of patient self-care in racial and ethnic differences has not been clearly established.

One needs to attend, to begin with, to differences across specific diseases or conditions. Psychosis and substance abuse, for instance, are related to contrasting differences. Blacks with psychotic disorders visit psychiatrists less often than whites. But blacks with substance abuse disorders have more psychiatric visits than whites (Kales et al., 2000). Other factors, from socioeconomic status to differences in cultural beliefs relating to fatalism

(Nelson et al., 2002) also complicate the picture. In addition, blacks and Hispanics are reported to distrust health care providers and expect discriminatory treatment more often than whites (LaVeist et al., 2000; Lillie-Blanton et al., 2000), but whether this affects their acceptance of recommended treatments or compliance with prescribed regimens has not been clearly demonstrated.

NEEDED RESEARCH

Improvements in health care by themselves are unlikely to either eliminate social inequalities in health or achieve optimal levels of population health (House and Williams, 2000; Kaplan et al., 2000).

Some evidence indicates that medical care explains only 10 percent of variation in adult mortality (U.S. Department of Health, Education, and Welfare, 1979), which has led to the widely held view that medical care makes a limited contribution to population differences in health status (Adler et al., 1993). However, medical care may have a greater effect on the health status of vulnerable populations, such as racial and ethnic minorities and low-status groups among older adults, than on the population in general (Williams, 1990). What this effect could be, what differences actually exist beyond those now documented, how they interact with multiple vulnerabilities in the older population, and how health care should be properly structured to address differences are all issues that require attention.

Research Need 14: Identify differences in health care—access, use, and quality—for racial and ethnic minority populations other than blacks.

To date, most research on differences in care has focused on blacks and whites, partly reflecting the absence in the Medicare file of high-quality ethnic identifiers for other groups. The few studies that have identified differences in quality and intensity of care for other groups leave the extent of the differences faced by Hispanics, American Indians and Alaska Natives, and Asians unclear (Institute of Medicine, 2002).

Research Need 15: Determine the reasons for differences in health care quality, focusing on the contributions of geographic variation, characteristics of health care institutions, provider behavior and stereotypes, and patient adherence to recommendations for care.

Multiple factors are almost certainly involved, as they are with differences in health outcomes, and need to be assessed against each other. Medical care may vary because of the health needs of different groups, or the types of care they seek, prefer, or can afford, or because of insurance coverage, provider behavior, or the policies and procedures of hospitals and health systems. Research attention is desirable across multiple dimensions of health care.

Geographic Variation Why care varies across areas is poorly understood. Some variation may be due to less adequate services in poor areas that are predominantly minority. However, geographic variation that is not rooted in any racial or ethnic factor could still produce racial and ethnic differences in care. Different ways to define geographic areas, different patterns across areas for various medical procedures, and the complex and changing settlement patterns for racial and ethnic groups all complicate the research challenge.

Health Care Institutions The specific characteristics of health care institutions and systems that affect racial and ethnic differences in care require attention. Financial, structural, and institutional factors need consideration, taking into account features of medical procedures, such as their cost, and the degree to which medical consensus exists about particular treatments.

Provider Behavior and Stereotypes Whether, and if so how, provider decisions about treatment are influenced by stereotypes requires consideration. Negative stereotypes and the unrecognized discrimination connected with them could contribute to systematic bias in the delivery of medical care. Evidence that this actually happens, and that medical decisions are sometimes inappropriate for this reason, does not exist.

Patient Compliance Racial and ethnic differences in acceptance of therapies and compliance with prescribed regimens deserve clarification. Differences across groups are unclear and may depend on the specific medical conditions, procedures, and prescriptions. The reasons for any differences also require study—whether they are due to differences in the way patients are treated or advised, in the cultural background of each patient, or in other factors.

11

The Life Course

Some racial and ethnic health differences are consistent across the age range, appearing among younger as well as older people. This consistency suggests that early life conditions could be important for late-life differences and that understanding the relative health status of racial and ethnic groups in late life may require study of health factors, including all the factors just discussed, at younger ages. The empirical evidence that late-life differences develop from events at earlier ages is scattered and uneven. Some evidence is indeed fairly strong, but much of it is largely suggestive and requires further confirmation.

Depending on the severity of their effects on health, early life events could produce later differences in three ways. First, if these events lead to some risk of early death, it could affect the eventual composition of cohorts of the aged of different racial and ethnic groups. The survivors in each group may be selected in different ways, producing differences in health status. Such selection processes are discussed above; to fully understand them would require a comprehensive investigation of the life course, beginning at the earliest ages.

Second, early life events may impair health, or alternatively lead to more robust health, and so confer permanent disadvantages or advantages or possibly a chronic risk of illness. Injuries that produce permanent disability, for instance, obviously have lifetime implications. Illness or malnutrition may affect the normal physiology and functioning of vital organs in a permanent way. If the immediate health effects are reversible, they may still leave someone more susceptible to later illness. For instance, impaired fetal development of the respiratory system could lead to greater susceptibility to chronic obstructive respiratory disease (Ben-Shlomo and Kuh, 2002).

Third, early life events may somehow set one on a pathway that results, possibly many years later, in impaired—or enhanced—health (Hertzman, 2004). Such experiences as early schooling may not immediately affect health but may decisively influence one's eventual level of completed education and foreclose certain career paths, affecting experiences and later behavior in ways that eventually affect health. For instance, nutritional deficiencies related to poverty, even if they have no irreversible health effect, may produce lung function deficiencies that in the long run result in greater susceptibility to infections of the upper respiratory system. Pathways may involve cumulative effects but are not determinate, since health and development are subject to many influences. The plasticity of these relations means that a person's late-life health status is not certain but depends on numerous contingencies (Rutter, 1996).

EARLY HEALTH DISADVANTAGE

Health in early life differs among racial and ethnic groups. Time trends since 1950 in birthweight and infant mortality—two basic though not necessarily the most appropriate indicators (Barker, 1998)—show consistent differences that favor whites over blacks and American Indians and Alaska Natives. For Asians and Hispanics, the contrasts with whites are less consistent, but they indicate that these minorities fare better with respect to birthweight though not, in the case of Hispanics, infant mortality. Little is known, however, about racial and ethnic differences in exposure to and experience with illnesses in early life.

Do the early life health differences that are known account for some portion of health and mortality differences among racial and ethnic groups at older ages? Although no coherent body of research attempts to assess such influences in comparison with contemporaneous or other explanations of differences, there is important research on the mechanisms by which early life environments may affect later health.

Conditions *in utero* and during the first year of life modify patterns of brain tissue growth and thereby alter the functioning of one or more neurophysiological centers of hormonal balance and activation. This functioning influences cellular growth, tissue development, and the ultimate physiological status and functioning of key organs, such as the heart, lungs, and kidneys. Ultimately affected are immune status, resilience, frailty, individual choices, and behavior (Hertzman et al., 2002). That early life health status has such long-term effects is demonstrated in some studies (Barker, 1998; Ben-Shlomo and Smith, 1991), though not all (Christensen et al., 1995; Leon, 1995; Vagero and Leon, 1994).

Consequences of early events and conditions may be lifelong or long delayed. Such early onset illnesses as schizophrenia and epilepsy (West, 1991), the complications generated by rheumatoid fever (Barker, 1998; Elo and Preston, 1992), injuries due to violence, and impairments caused by substance abuse lead to proximate shifts in individuals' health and mortality risks that endure for a lifetime. In contrast, impaired placental development, poor maternal nutrition, and extreme low birthweight may have effects not seen for a long time; all are suspected to be implicated in the late onset of coronary heart disease, non-insulin-dependent diabetes, lung disease, chronic bronchitis, and reduced immunocompetence (Barker, 1998; Chandra et al., 1989; Fall et al., 1998; Lucas, 1991, 1994; Lucas et al., 1999; Thurlbeck, 1992; Vagero and Leon, 1994). Similarly, early nutritional status may compromise later health status (Smith and Kuh, 1997).

The health effects of early events may not be immediately visible. For instance, there is early evidence of a link between early educational attainment and avoidance of cognitive decline late in life. This link could be due to synaptic connections in the brain, providing a cognitive reserve generated by education itself, or by higher levels of cognitive stimulation, or to the beneficial impact of higher self-esteem among the more educated (Hertzman et al., 2002; Manly and Mayeux, 2004). Similarly, the effects of stress may not be visible early in life. Although stress and resulting allostatic load have been investigated mainly in adults, it is possible that losses of plasticity of physiological response that increase the risk of chronic conditions could also be related to nonoptimal exposures to stress early in life (Hertzman et al., 2002).

PATHWAYS TO DISADVANTAGE

Early health disadvantage may be compounded if individuals are put on pathways that, whatever their immediate affect on health, lead to poorer health later on. Research suggests that black children experience higher levels of poverty, more limited educational experiences, and more disruptive home lives—in segregated neighborhoods or with single mothers or unemployed parents. Such conditions constitute possible pathways to later health disadvantage.

Evidence regarding such pathways has accumulated slowly. The causative processes involved are complex, not readily amenable to representation in simple models, and often impossible to test without exceedingly rich information that spans the life of at least one cohort. Various dimensions of early environments can put one on a pathway, and only a few have been studied.

One important dimension is the socioeconomic status of the family of origin that may shape early life through numerous mediating mechanisms.

Some research has focused directly on the effects of early childhood status and deprivation on late adult health and mortality (Ben-Shlomo and Kuh, 1997; Ben-Shlomo and Smith, 1991; Blackwell et al., 2000; Felitti et al., 1998; Forsdahl, 1978, 2002; Hayward and Gorman, 2002; Moore et al., 1997; Power et al., 1990, 1998; Rahkonen et al., 1997; Wadsworth, 1991; Wadsworth and Kuh, 1997). Few such studies focus on ethnic and racial differences in the processes involved (Doblhammer, 2002; Warner and Hayward, 2002). Few studies also attempt to identify mediating mechanisms, which are important because low socioeconomic status is not itself a disease nor intrinsically tied to poorer health.

One possible mediating mechanism is access to and use of health care. Differences in health care between white and minority children and their mothers have been documented (Institute of Medicine, 2002). This may be relevant to late-life health status and mortality, though the effects of prenatal care on fetal growth and birthweight are now in dispute. The relevance of other aspects of health care—less use of prescribed medications, fewer visits to physicians, poorer compliance with vaccination schedules—has not been confirmed.

Another mediating mechanism, much more complex and virtually unexplored, involves the mutual dependence of health and socioeconomic status (discussed earlier as a possible selection process). If impoverished early environments are associated with worse health, this may limit one's opportunities in life, which in turn may expose one to greater health risks. Health differences in adulthood could be exacerbated by such a mechanism. Some research has attempted to model the influences involved (Palloni and Milesi, 2002; Power et al., 1986), and other research has sought to determine the magnitude of the effects (Hack et al., 2002; Lundberg, 1991; Nystrom Peck, 1992; Nystrom Peck and Lundberg, 1995; Nystrom Peck and Vagero, 1987; Power et al., 1990; Wadsworth, 1986). But these efforts have met only limited success (Palloni and Milesi, 2002), and the skeptical tone of early evaluations is still appropriate today (Blane et al., 1993). The extent to which such a mechanism may account for racial and ethnic differences is unknown.

Other features of early environments that may put individuals on pathways to disadvantage include exposure to discrimination or stigmatization (as discussed above), the physical and social isolation of a group, and exposure to conflict and violence. Some research suggests that stressful events, more commonly experienced in deprived social environments, lead to poor maternal health and increase the risks of fetal underdevelopment and low birthweight (Hogue and Hargraves, 1993; Williams and Collins, 1995; Zambrana et al., 1997). Evidence from animal and human studies shows that infants subjected to abuse, lack of parental care, and, more generally, higher levels of violence and hostility experience physiological changes in hormonal regulatory mechanisms, changes that are precursors of and a predisposition to various chronic conditions (Bornstein and Cote, 2001; Coe, 1999; Francis et al., 1999; Hertzman et al., 2002). Experiencing certain environments may "mark" individuals—perhaps through a number of physiological imprinting mechanisms—in ways that could increase the risk of later morbidity.

Understanding the implications of early life events, as well as of events over the life course, may in some cases require a focus on health in late life or even at the oldest ages. People who live to extremely old ages tend to remain healthy and functional much longer than others (Hitt et al., 1999). Expanding knowledge of the extremely long-lived population holds special significance for racial and ethnic minorities. For instance, the Hispanic paradox—the better health of Hispanics relative to better-off whites (Franzini et al., 2001)—raises the question of whether there is a robust aging minority population that might reward study.

NEEDED RESEARCH

Improving understanding of the consequences of early experiences for differences in adult health and mortality is a complex task. Several inter-related types of work are needed. First, research is needed to identify key early experiences and the precise mediating mechanisms through which they affect later health. Though some important factors have been identified, more work needs to be done. Also needed is better understanding of the conditions that enhance or inhibit the effects of such factors. Second, research is needed to better document racial and ethnic differences in these early experiences. Only limited and superficial evidence on this is now available. Third, research is needed to determine whether the effects of early experiences and initial differences in them actually account for some portion of racial and ethnic differences at older ages. This issue remains unexplored.

Research Need 16: Place particular emphasis on panel studies that follow cohorts over time in order to study differences in health among racial and ethnic groups over the life course.

Such panel studies should include physiological and psychological measures as well as assessments of environmental conditions. Some such studies are in progress, following British and Canadian cohorts (Hertzman et al., 2002; Wadsworth, 1991). Other large longitudinal studies of somewhat different design, such as the National Longitudinal Survey of Youth (NLSY) and the Panel Study of Income Dynamics in the United States and a survey like the NLSY in Canada can be used for partial tests of some hypotheses. One convenient way to produce panel data might be to follow up on previously surveyed samples, such as those for other National Longitudinal Surveys, on young women, mature women, young men, and older men, even though some of the surveys have been previously discontinued. Two other longitudinal studies—the Coronary Artery Risk Development in Young Adults study and the Atherosclerosis Risk in Communities study—include, by design, samples of whites and black, and may therefore be particularly useful for looking at racial differences.

Short of cohort studies, various other approaches can be taken to analyze life course influences. Surveys of adult health could be enhanced with information about childhood experiences. Retrospective questions could be used, though they are subject to recall bias, and responses can be distorted because of current status. Data can sometimes be obtained from administrative records matched with individual survey records. For instance, birth records contain information on birthweight that could be added to a number of ongoing surveys. Similarly, school records may contain information of past illnesses or health-related events (prolonged absences, personality reports, etc.). Test scores and examination results could also be useful to roughly characterize the school environment of survey respondents. A further possible approach is to extend existing data sets by linking them with other data sources. All these approaches require interdisciplinary teams and close collaboration among funding agencies, some of which may support work on early childhood and others on adult health and mortality. There are also obviously difficult issues of methodology and data quality, problems with releasing sufficient data to allow matching, and issues of confidentiality that must be attended to in each case.

Studies could also focus on specific stages of the life course to document the operation of mechanisms that are hypothesized to mediate the effects of early experiences on adult health. If deprivation alters key physiological parameters during early childhood, it should be possible to verify this effect without a longitudinal study. Uncovering such effects is crucial to any argument that early experiences affect adult health through physiological programming or imprinting. Studies of these mechanisms may require invasive procedures (such as extensive and expensive blood tests, magnetic resonance imaging, etc.) but could be completed relatively quickly. For instance, studies could focus on metabolic variables among younger individuals exposed or not exposed to known sources of stress to determine allostatic load and to assess whether physiological plasticity of response can be lost at early ages, and, if so, with what consequences.

Studies that combine data sets covering different stages in the life course would be useful to draw inferences across life stages. With properly designed estimation (and simulation) procedures, composite data sets would allow reasonable inferences about a range of early exposure effects and about their importance relative to contemporaneous determinants of health.

Besides attending to early stages in the life course, late stages might also receive some attention. Minority older adults who are exceptionally healthy might provide clues to appropriate behavior modification strategies to decrease mortality and morbidity across the lifespan. The Macarthur Successful Aging Cohort study covers whites and some blacks, but the superior health status of other racial and ethnic minorities, despite poorer socioeconomic status, suggests that they should be included in studies.

Whether implementing cohort studies or other approaches, social scientists and epidemiologists need to pay more attention to and collaborate more closely with those carrying out studies with animal models to learn about the plausible operation, boundaries, and reach of biological effects. Some of the most important work on the effects of early experiences on adult health status has been inspired by studies with monkeys and rats. Similarly, a remarkable number of studies relating early deprivation to physiological imprinting are based on animal models (Barker, 1998).

12

Interventions

Racial and ethnic differences in late-life health may reflect the disadvantaged status of some groups and reinforce their disadvantage. Some health differences may also reflect unequal treatment. It is reasonable for society to assign some priority to interventions to reduce health differences, and this chapter considers the evidence on the effects of intervention.

The goal of reducing differences needs to be carefully defined. What is of interest is improving group health, reducing differences without impairing the health of other groups. Interventions that improve health overall while possibly exacerbating differences should be considered, especially if the effect on differences is temporary, but they need to be assessed against other, neutral or differential-reducing interventions. It is important to recall that the health differences we consider involve groups, not individuals, though our focus is on interventions that improve individual health. Researchers need to be aware of events that could affect group differences simply by altering group membership—by facilitating return migration of ill elderly immigrants, for instance, which would have an effect on group differences.

We consider interventions in two categories: specific, directed interventions to change behavior and broader policy changes that may also have behavioral effects.

CHANGING INDIVIDUAL BEHAVIOR

Interventions to promote behavior change can play a role in improving health at older ages. Whether they can also contribute to reducing racial and ethnic differences in health is less certain, and it may depend not just on the particular interventions, but also on their specific design, targeting, and implementation. We consider the role of health promotion at older ages and then touch briefly on its possible effect on differences, about which little research has been done.

Health Promotion at Older Ages

Health promotion can make a difference in the care of older persons. Some health care providers are trained to counsel older persons to stop smoking, moderate their alcohol use, exercise, and lose weight. Older persons on their own sometimes attempt to improve their health by modifying behavior, making choices about medical care, or using complementary or alternative therapies.

Health promotion interventions take place in a complex environment that includes family and social relationships, economic and geographic factors, and physical barriers and opportunities, all of which influence older persons' ability to process health information and translate it into new behavior. Furthermore, outcomes are also influenced by how individuals choose to incorporate health promotion ideas that may reach them, with various levels of accuracy, from various sources. Cultural factors may also modify individual responses.

Health promotion may be more effective with older than younger people, who may be more willing to adopt healthy life-styles (Stewart et al., 2001). To reduce the incidence of diabetes, Knowler et al. (2002) found that a life-style intervention was superior to Metformin (a drug which keeps the liver from making too much sugar), with the life-style intervention being particularly effective in an older age group. Likewise, Appel et al. (2001) showed that hypertension could be reduced in a cohort of older persons through a 9-month sodium intervention. There may be important differences between younger and older persons in how they respond to health promotion activities.

The focus of health promotion in later life is different than at younger ages. For those over age 65, the focus is primarily to reduce age-associated morbidity and disability and the effects of cumulative disease comorbidities. For instance, the Fitness Arthritis in Seniors Trial achieved a significant reduction in disability and an improvement in physical performance in an older cohort despite having no effect on the actual disease process (Ettinger et al., 1997). In the over-85 age group, health promotion focuses almost exclusively on maintaining function and enhancing the quality of life.

Possible Effects on Differences

Health promotion could have different effects for various racial and ethnic groups. We illustrate possible reasons for this, though the research on each is not conclusive.

First, racial and ethnic groups may differ initially on the behavior that one seeks to influence. As discussed above, some unhealthy behaviors are more characteristic of older whites—smoking, less frequent Pap tests and mammogram screening—and others are more characteristic of older blacks and Hispanics—less physical activity and obesity (Winkleby and Cubbin, 2004). The relative physical inactivity of blacks and Mexican Americans cannot be explained by the socioeconomic status of individuals (Crespo et al., 2000). Also, even at similar socioeconomic levels, Mexican American women have more body fat than white women of similar body mass (Casas et al., 2001). (There is more limited information on these behaviors for Asians and American Indians and Alaska Natives.) It is reasonable to expect that health promotion interventions targeted at specific behaviors should have differential effects across groups, but whether those with more or less healthy behavioral profiles would be more affected is undetermined.

Second, some interventions may affect socioeconomic groups differently, with some being more responsive to them because of differences in education or income. Some interventions, such as smoking cessation, have been more successful among more educated people, but others, such as cholesterol screening, appear to affect socioeconomic groups equally (Cutler, 2004). Since racial and ethnic groups differ in socioeconomic status, interventions with disproportionate influence on higher status groups could affect differences, increasing the black disadvantage but reducing the Asian advantage (and the Hispanic advantage for mortality) relative to whites. Particularly if such effects are temporary, this difference is not necessarily a reason for avoiding such interventions.

Third, the social situation for members of some racial or ethnic groups may favor a stronger or weaker response to a specific intervention. The social environment plays a large role in the health of older persons, with younger family members involved in caregiving to maintain the health of older persons and keep them in their home environment. Extended caregiving networks are reported to be more active among some racial and ethnic minorities than others (Navaie-Waliser et al., 2001; Roth et al., 2001; Williams and Dilworth-Anderson, 2002). Eyler et al. (1999) found that, in comparison with black and American Indian women, Hispanic women were more likely to have high levels of social support, which promoted physical activity. The amount of social support, including also support from the wider community, may determine whether health promotion succeeds or fails. Support, however, is double-edged: it can also reinforce opposition to behavioral change.

Fourth, some groups may react more positively, for cultural reasons, to particular types of interventions, as can be seen for the use of alternative therapies (Jones, 2001; Loera et al., 2001). Hispanic and Asian older adults use both folk medicine and Western medicine, depending on the illness and symptoms, as well as their ability to obtain traditional health care (AppleWhite, 1995; Torsch and Ma, 2000). Despite the heavy promotion of alternative therapies and their common use by older adults, such therapies are inadequately studied. If they have any effect, they could produce health differences. The effect could also be negative, in deterring or delaying the search for more effective therapies. Not only healthy behaviors are promoted. Nutritional supplements that may or may not be useful are also promoted, as more broadly, are such unhealthful behaviors as smoking and the consumption of fast food. Racial and ethnic groups differ in such behaviors, but what role promotion plays and how best to communicate opposing messages to particular groups is unknown.

NEEDED RESEARCH

Given how little is known with any certainty about the effects of health promotion interventions on racial and ethnic differences, fairly basic research issues need to be addressed. What health care seeking behavior is typical of different groups is probably the place to start.

Research Need 17: Measure the use of complementary and alternative therapies by racial and ethnic groups.

How are these therapies incorporated into self treatment? Do these therapies have any substantial health effect, and how do they affect quality of life? The answers to such questions may provide guides for the design of health promotion interventions.

Subsequently, research could proceed to identify the appropriate health care seeking behavior and risk behaviors to target across different ethnic groups. Information is limited on the prevalence of health risk behaviors in older cohorts, especially Asian and American Indian and Alaska Native populations. Reliable information on obesity, diet, and sedentary life-style patterns would allow for a better understanding of how these risks affect morbidity and functional disability in these populations. Better information would help guide the selection of interventions and the selection of target groups in the population.

Some research could also be directed at understanding differential responses to health promotion by age, socioeconomic status, and racial and ethnic group. Health promotion strategies that succeed in one population may not be successful in another. The evidence that older cohorts respond better than younger cohorts is intriguing, but it requires confirmation and explanation. The evidence of differential response by education also needs study: How should interventions be designed to more effectively reach less educated, lower income groups? Racial and ethnic differences in response to interventions need to be identified and explained: Are they due to socio-economic factors, to differences in the support environment, to particular cultural traits, or to some combination of these factors?

SOCIAL POLICY

Direct promotion of individual behavior change is only one of the tools available to reduce health disadvantages among particular racial and ethnic groups. The range of possible interventions to achieve such public health objectives includes

• economic incentives and disincentives linked to health-relevant behaviors;
• changes in the informational environment—education, product labeling, and regulation of commercial speech;
• direct regulation through penalties for behavior risky to oneself or others or for organizations that fail to deliver contracted health benefits;
• indirect regulation through the legal tort system; and
• deregulatory actions that dismantle legal barriers to desired public health behaviors (Gostin, 2001).

Such measures can be designed to affect personal behavior (through education, incentives, or penalties) or to work indirectly: through modifying the general environment for behavior or through affecting health care providers or other producers of relevant products and services (Sampson and Morenoff, 2001).

Effectiveness of Interventions

Relatively little is known about how interventions affect health differences. In fact, their effectiveness at improving population health, regardless of their effect on differences, is still a matter for discussion. Large-scale community experiments aimed at changing behavior in the population at large (not just among older adults) have been disappointing. Multifaceted community intervention experiments that promoted healthy behaviors have shown some effects, such as those in the 12,866-subject experiment labeled

MRFIT (Multiple Risk Factor Intervention Trial Research Group, 1982, 1990, 1996). However, changes were modest, and control groups showed similar outcomes (Cutler, 2004; Syme, 2002).

In contrast, some health risk behaviors have changed over time, and public interventions seem to have played an important role: an example is smoking. National cigarette consumption per capita reached its peak in the early 1960s. Since the 1964 Surgeon General's report on the dangers of smoking (U.S. Department of Health, Education, and Welfare, 1964), consumption has steadily dropped to less than half the peak level, declining roughly in parallel among whites and blacks. Standing by itself, the Surgeon General's report would probably not have generated such a wide-ranging and sustained response. But the report did not stand by itself. It mobilized public opinion and eventually generated a variety of legislative responses, including taxes on cigarettes, restrictions on broadcast advertising, anti-tobacco advertising campaigns, limits on access to cigarettes, and bans on smoking in various establishments and public places.

Antismoking policies have been extensively studied (Chaloupka and Warner, 2000; U.S. Department of Health and Human Services, 2000); as summarized by Cutler (2004), many of them are effective. Generally, a 10 percent increase in prices (through taxation, for instance) reduces consumption of cigarettes by 4 percent, with young men affected more than young women (Chaloupka and Pacula, 1998) and the poor affected substantially more than the rich (Gruber and Kosygi, 2002). Antitobacco advertising can have large effects: California's $26 million media campaign of the early 1990s reduced smoking by an average (per year) of eight packs per person. Workplace smoking bans reduce the number of workers smoking by 5 percent and also reduce consumption among workers who continue to smoke (Cutler, 2004). Such policy changes, while effective, are nevertheless insufficient to account for the overall historical reduction in smoking, which must reflect, in addition, a broad-based movement away from smoking among millions of people. Somehow, in the late 20th century, the political timing was right for antitobacco measures, and growing public approval helped make them effective.

Blacks have benefited as much or slightly more than whites from smoking declines over the last four decades. The same cannot be said across education groups. Smokers among high school dropouts were 6 percentage points more numerous than among college graduates in 1966, and 19 percentage points more numerous in 1995.

When promotion of health behavior becomes part of a broad social movement, involving and mobilizing a range of social actors—national and local legislators, the media, private business, volunteer groups, etc.—wide-ranging effects such as those from antismoking campaigns are possible. Cutler (2004) refers to this phenomenon as permeation, the saturation of

the environment with informational messages, including and perhaps especially messages from one's peers. The same phenomenon arguably has been
at work in the reduction in drunk driving since the early 1980s, spurred by
the activities of Mothers Against Drunk Driving and other grassroots programs.

One factor that has helped keep campaigns against smoking and drunk
driving going has been the presence of externalities, the argument that
others are hurt when people smoke or drive drunk (Cutler, 2004; Warner,
2001). In contrast, this argument has not been prominent so far in attempts
to reduce obesity and has not been sufficient in the public debate about
guns. Campaigns also have costs, of course. In addition to the resources
needed for intervention, there are the burdens, difficult to quantify, that
may be imposed on individual behavior, as when smokers are required to
limit where they smoke (Gostin, 2001; Warner, 2001).

Targeted Interventions

If whites and minorities benefit equally from society-wide interventions, there would appear to be little reason to target interventions to
particular groups. However, interventions do not necessarily have the same
effect across racial and ethnic groups. For instance, long-term declines in
smoking, roughly similar among whites and blacks, were paralleled among
Hispanics and Asian and Pacific Islanders, but at somewhat lower levels,
while declines were much more limited among American Indians and Alaska
Natives. Particular subgroups among these minorities—reproductive-age
American Indian women and Southeast Asian men, for instance, show
strikingly high tobacco use (U.S. Department of Health and Human Services,
1998). Aside from smoking policy, quite different types of health policies,
such as changes in health care regulation and funding, could also have
disparate effects.

Are targeted interventions ever worth consideration? They raise various
concerns relating to equity (Hudson, 2002). To the extent that federal
social policy has increasingly benefited the aged, what effects have there
been on equity across age groups (Meyers and Darity, 2000; Preston, 1984)?
What resources are appropriate to address the special needs of particular
immigrant groups among the aged, in comparison with groups that have
spent their entire lives in the United States (Jasso et al., 2004)? How can one
think about the fairness of the distribution of scarce national resources that
do not provide broad assistance across the entire population but may be
effective in addressing the needs of particular groups? These are broad
philosophical and legal questions that are central in the history of the
country's public policy making and its democratic ideals (Gostin, 2001).

There are two approaches that largely avoid these difficult equity issues. A simple approach is to build on the fact that racial and ethnic groups differ in their health problems, as already observed. Focusing on some health problems rather than others, even if no particular groups are targeted, would have a differential effect. Devoting more resources to diabetes, in particular, would probably benefit blacks, Hispanics, and American Indians more than whites or Asians, if the interventions are effective. This approach requires that all groups be reached equally and that the intervention effects do not differ by economic status, important assumptions that cannot be taken for granted. Similarly, programs to improve hospital quality are likely to reduce black-white differences in care to the extent blacks go to poorer quality hospitals, as could efforts to direct patients to better quality hospitals (Skinner et al., 2003).

A second approach comes from noting other differences between racial and ethnic groups. They may react differently to interventions, and some degree of specificity may be appropriate in order to reach members of particular groups. Health motivations, and resulting health-seeking behavior, could vary. While long life is presumably an important personal goal for everyone, the emphasis on it may differ for groups who suffer a multitude of environmental and life stressors (Baum, 2001). Cultural and socio-economic considerations may influence the perceptions, experiences, and expression of health and illness (Dilworth-Anderson and Gibson, 2002; Goldman and Smith, 2002). For example, for those groups with relatively low life expectancy, quality of life may be a more important consideration than longevity. Thus, interventions that focus on promoting life extension may not be as effective as those that target quality of life.

Similarly, interventions that focus on the personal consequences of behavior may be less effective, for some groups, than those that focus on significant others who may be affected (Warner, 2001). For instance, behavioral interventions directed at the wives of men who have had a heart attack may be more effective, for some groups, than those directed at the men themselves (Taylor et al., 1985).

Finally, different racial and ethnic groups may show age-related changes at different times and to different degrees (Crimmins et al., 2004). Treatment may therefore be more effective at different ages for different groups; for instance, bone density testing at younger ages for white and Asian women in comparison with Hispanic and black women, mammograms at younger ages for black women, and blood pressure screening at younger ages for black men than other groups.

Indirect Effects of Policy

The policy possibilities we have considered are limited in an important respect. A broader conception of the possibilities would include any government measure that results in some transfer of resources, as well as other government regulations that, intentionally or not, affect health differences or the factors underlying them. Though such policies may be adopted for reasons unrelated to health, they may have important indirect effects on health differences.

Since socioeconomic factors have an important relationship to health differences, any program that affects resource distribution in the society could have health implications. For instance, changes in Medicare funding could affect health differences. As noted above, exclusive dependence on Medicare is higher among Hispanics and blacks than among whites, so that changes in the program could have more effects on them. Given the known and hypothesized effects on health in late life of childhood conditions, one may consider racial and ethnic differences in the socioeconomic conditions of childhood and government programs that exacerbate those effects or do not attempt to remedy them (Warner and Hayward, 2002).

Changes in immigration regulations could also affect health differences, by affecting the number, selectivity, or experience of the recent immigrants who constitute an important proportion of some racial and ethnic groups. Tighter controls on immigration, for instance, could increase the risks that illegal immigrants take, reduce the propensity for circular migration and therefore modify salmon bias (the return to their native countries of ill immigrants), and make immigrants a more select group in ways that could have unpredictable implications for population health.

National policy may in fact have had substantial influence on health differences from the 1960s to the 1990s. From 1968 to 1978, blacks showed larger gains than whites in life expectancy and larger declines in mortality rates from a variety of causes (Cooper et al., 1981). But from 1980 to 1991, the black-white gap in health status widened, whether measured by life expectancy, excess deaths, or infant mortality (National Center for Health Statistics, 1994; Williams and Collins, 1995), before narrowing again in the 1990s. The trends in the mortality gap also appeared at older ages, among those aged 65-74 (National Center for Health Statistics, 2003). The narrowing of the gap in the late 1960s and the early 1970s coincided roughly with gains from the civil rights movement and a parallel narrowing in the income gap between blacks and whites (Economic Report of the President, 1998; Williams, 2001a). The reversal of the trend in health differences beginning around 1980 coincided with substantial changes in national social and economic policies, during which the health status of economically vulnerable populations worsened in several states (Lurie et al., 1984; Mandinger, 1985). What influence on health differences was actually exerted by national policy, by economic gains, or by the empowerment and increasing social acceptance of blacks are obviously research questions of interest.

When considering public health measures targeted at reducing racial or ethnic health disadvantage, therefore, one should keep in mind the ways in which other government actions, taken for a variety of extraneous reasons, can also affect racial and ethnic differences, supporting or possibly undermining measures directed at improving health.

NEEDED RESEARCH

Much is obviously not known about the policy possibilities for dealing with racial and ethnic differences in late-life health. There is a need to examine the effects of broad social policies on a wide variety of health behaviors among older people of different racial and ethnic groups. The effects of specific policies, such as taxation, also require corraboration for various population groups, such as recent immigrants (Jasso et al., 2004). A simple distinction between whites and minority groups is clearly insufficient in assessing differential effects. More broadly, there appears to be little analysis of the differential effects of interventions at the individual, community, or national levels by age and race or ethnicity (Emmons, 2001). There may be large cohort or period influences that would make public policies more or less effective for different groups at different times (Warner, 2001). Analysis should use as much existing data as possible, but it may be hampered by the lack of good, representative data, especially for older adults and recent immigrants.

Research Need 18: Characterize long-term trends (and possible lags) in the effects of changing social policy—federal, state, and local—on health differences and on public health.

For instance, popular expectations may have been too high that the 1964 civil rights laws, which marked a significant public policy change, would have large and immediate effects on the health and well-being of that generation of blacks. Much time was required to prepare regulations to implement legislation—to change the nature of segregated health care facilities, to improve the availability of good prenatal care and well-baby check-ups, to expand the possibilities for better jobs, and to improve environmental and housing conditions. Overcoming long-term neglect and lack of access are long-term projects that are still in process. How lags in the effects of public policy differentially affect racial and ethnic groups at different points in the life course requires sustained scrutiny (Hudson, 2002; Warner, 2001).

This research issue also has a prospective dimension. As policy options and interventions are developed to deal with current major issues in public health, research is needed of the ways in which these policies and interventions may affect racial and ethnic groups differently. The epidemic of obesity, for instance, is commanding increasing public and professional attention. Researchers need to attend to the mechanisms of influence of legal interventions and the ways they may have differential effects (Emmons, 2001; Gostin, 2001; Warner, 2001). For instance, one possible reason for the limited progress that has been made to combat obesity, particularly among the disadvantaged, may have to do with the price structure for various foods. If a premium must be paid for lean meats, reduced fat, and low-calorie foods, availability and consumption of these will be more limited at lower socioeconomic levels, with possible differential effects across racial and ethnic groups. When combined with cultural food patterns, the wide availability of high-starch and high-fat food stuffs, lack of leisure time opportunities, limited leisure time outlets, and the cheap, sedentary entertainment of television, public policies to affect health behaviors face difficult barriers (Warner, 2001).

One option, requiring special research attention, is supplementing universal health intervention policies with policies targeted at specific groups (Syme, 2002). Universal health policies (e.g., Medicare and Medicaid) are reported to have improved the health of blacks and other disproportionately low-income groups (Meyers and Darity, 2000). Whether some targeting of interventions would be useful to reduce group health disadvantages is worth investigation (Hudson, 2002; Syme, 2002).

References

Abraido-Lanza AF, Dohrenwend BP, Ng-Mak DS, Turner JB. 1999. The Latino mortality paradox: A test of the "salmon bias" and healthy migrant hypotheses. *American Journal of Public Health* 89(10):1543-1548.

Adams P, Hurd M, McFadden D, Merrill A, Ribeiro T. 2003. Healthy, wealthy, and wise? Tests for direct causal paths between health and socioeconomic status. *Journal of Econometrics* 112:3-56.

Adams-Campbell LL, Nwankwo M, Ukoli F, Omene J, Haile GT, Kuller LH. 1990. Body fat distribution patterns and blood pressure in black and white women. *Journal of the National Medical Association* 82:573-576.

Adler NE, Newman K. 2002. Socioeconomic disparities in health: Pathways and policies. *Health Affairs* 21(2):60-76.

Adler NE, Boyce WT, Chesney MA, Folkman S, Syme SL. 1993. Socioeconomic inequalities in health: No easy solution. *Journal of the American Medical Association* 269(24):3140-3145.

Adler NE, Boyce T, Chesney M, Cohen S, Folkman S, Kahn RL, Syme SL. 1994. Socioeconomic status and health: The challenge of the gradient. *American Psychologist* 49(1):15-24.

Albert MS, Jones K, Savage CR, Berkman L, Seeman T, Blazer D, Rowe JW. 1995. Predictors of cognitive change in older persons: MacArthur Studies of Successful Aging. *Psychology and Aging* 10:578-589.

Alexis M, Haines GH, Simon LS. 1980. *Black Consumer Profiles*. Ann Arbor, MI: Division of Research, Graduate School of Business Administration, University of Michigan.

Allen TW. 1994. *The Invention of the White Race: Racial Oppression and Social Control*. New York: Verso Books.

Allison DB, Gallagher D, Heo M, Pi-Sunyer FX, Heymsfield SB. 1997. Body mass index and all-cause mortality among people age 70 and over: The Longitudinal Study of Aging. *International Journal of Obesity* 21(6):424-431.

Allport GW. 1958. *The Nature of Prejudice*. Reading, MA: Addison-Wesley.

Amaro H, Russo NF, Johnson J. 1987. Family and work predictors of psychological well-being among Hispanic women professionals. *Psychology of Women Quarterly* 11:505-521.

Amick BC III, McDonough P, Chang H, Rogers WH, Pieper CF, Duncan G. 2002. Relationship between all-cause mortality and cumulative working life course psychosocial and physical exposures in the United States Labor M꞉ ket from 1968 to 1992. *Psychosomatic Medicine* 64:1-12.

Anderson N. 1989. Racial differences in stress-induced cardiovascular reactivity and hypertension: Current status and substantive issues. *Psychological Bulletin* 105(1):89-105.

Anderson N. 1998. Levels of analysis in health science: A framework for integrating sociobehavioral and biomedical research. *Annals of the New York Academy of Sciences* 840:563-576.

Anderson NB. 1995. Behavioral and sociocultural perspectives on ethnicity and health: Introduction to the special issue. *Health Psychology* 14(7):589-591.

Anderson NB, Armstead CA. 1995. Toward understanding the association of socioeconomic status and health: A new challenge for the biopsychosocial approach. *Psychosomatic Medicine* 57:213-225.

Anderson RN. 2001. Deaths: Leading causes for 1999. *National Vital Statistics Reports* 49(11):1-87.

Anon. 2000. Census, race and science. *Nature Genetics* 24:97-98.

Anon. 2001. Genes, drugs and race. *Nature Genetics* 29:239-240.

Appel LJ, Espeland MA, Easter L, Wilson AC, Folmar S, Lacy CR. 2001. Effects of reduced sodium intake on hypertension control in older individuals. *Archives of Internal Medicine* 161:685-693.

AppleWhite SL. 1995. Curanderismo: Demystifying the health beliefs and practices of elderly Mexican Americans. *Health and Social Work* 20(4):247-253.

Armstead CA, Lawler KA, Gorden G, Cross J, Gibbons J. 1989. Relationship of racial stressors to blood pressure responses and anger expression in black college students. *Health Psychology* 8(5):541-556.

Armstrong LR, Hall HI, Wingo PA, Kassim S. 2002. Invasive cervical cancer among Hispanic and non-Hispanic women—United States, 1992-1999. *Morbidity and Mortality Weekly Report* 51(47):1067-1070.

Arozullah AM, Ferreira MR, Bennett RL, Gilman S, Henderson WG, Daley J, Khuri S, Bennett CL. 1999. Racial variation in the use of laparoscopic cholecystectomy in the Department of Veterans Affairs Medical System. *Journal of the American College of Surgeons* 188(6):604-622.

Bachrach C, McNicoll, G. 2003. Causal analysis in the population sciences: A symposium—Introduction. *Population and Development Review* 29(3):443-447.

Baillie GM, Sherer JT, Weart CW. 1998. Insulin and coronary artery disease: Is syndrome X the unifying hypothesis? *Annals of Pharmacotherapy* 32(2):233-247.

Baker DW, Stevens CD, Brook RH. 1996. Determinants of emergency department use: Are race and ethnicity important? *Annals of Emergency Medicine* 28(6):677-682.

Baldridge D. 2001. The elder population and long-term care. Pp. 137-164 in *Promises to Keep: Public Health Policy for American Indians and Alaska Natives in the 21st Century*. Dixon M, Roubideaux Y, eds. Washington, DC: American Public Health Association.

Barker DJP. 1998. *Mothers, Babies and Health in Later Life*. 2nd ed. Edinburgh: Churchill Livingstone.

Bassuk SS, Glass TA, Berkman LF. 1999. Social disengagement and incident cognitive decline in community-dwelling elderly persons. *Annals of Internal Medicine* 131(3):165-173.

Baum A. 2001. Behavioral and psychosocial intervention to modify pathophysiology and disease control. Pp. 450-488 in National Research Council, *Promoting Health: Intervention Strategies from Social and Behavioral Research*. Smedley BD, Syme SL, eds. Washington, DC: National Academy Press.

Been V. 1997. Coming to the nuisance or going to the barrios? A longitudinal analysis of environmental justice claims. *Ecology Law Quarterly* 24:1-56.

Ben-Shlomo Y, Kuh D. 1997. *A Life Course Approach to Chronic Disease Epidemiology*. New York: Oxford University Press.

Ben-Shlomo Y, Kuh D. 2002. A life course approach to chronic disease epidemiology: Conceptual models, empirical challenges and interdisciplinary perspectives. *International Journal of Epidemiology* 31:285-293.

Ben-Shlomo Y, Smith GD. 1991. Deprivation in infancy or in adult life: Which is more important for mortality risk? *Lancet* 337(8740).

Benner JS, Glynn RJ, Mogun H, Neumann PJ, Weinstein MC, Avorn J. 2002. Long-term persistence in use of statin therapy in elderly patients. *Journal of the American Medical Association* 288(4):455-461.

Berkman LF, Leo-Summers L, Horwitz RI. 1992. Emotional support and survival after myocardial infarction. A prospective, population-based study of the elderly. *Annals of Internal Medicine* 117:1003-1009.

Berkman LF, Blumenthal J, Burg M, Carney RM, Catellier D, Cowan MJ, Czajkowski SM, DeBusk R, Hosking J, Jaffe A, Kaufmann PG, Mitchell P, Norman J, Powell LH, Raczynski JM, Schneiderman N, Enhancing Recovery in Coronary Heart Disease Patients (ENRICHD) Investigators. 2003. Effects of treating depression and low perceived social support on clinical events after myocardial infarction: The Enhancing Recovery in Coronary Heart Disease Patients (ENRICHD) Randomized Trial. *Journal of the American Medical Association* 289(23):3106-3116.

Bigler RS, Avehart CJ, Liben LS. 2003. Race and the workforce: Occupational status, aspirations, and stereotyping among African American children. *Developmental Psychology* 39(3):572-580.

Bjorck JP, Lee YS, Cohen LH. 1997. Control beliefs and faith as stress moderators for Korean American versus Caucasian American Protestants. *American Journal of Community Psychology* 25(1):61-72.

Blackwell D, Hayward MD, Crimmins E. 2000. Does childhood health affect chronic morbidity in later life? *Social Science and Medicine* 52:1269-1284.

Blane D, Smith GD, M Bartley. 1993. Social selection: What does it contribute to social class differences in health? *Sociology of Health & Illness* 15(1).

Blendon R, Aiken L, Freeman H, Corey C. 1989. Access to medical care for black and white Americans. *Journal of the American Medical Association* 261:278-281.

Blumenthal JA, Jiang W, Waugh RA, Frid DJ, Morris JJ, Coleman RE, Hanson M, Babyak M, Thyrum ET, Krantz DS, O'Connor C. 1995. Mental stress-induced ischemia in the laboratory and ambulatory ischemia during daily life: Association and hemodynamic features. *Circulation* 92:2102-2108.

Bobak M, Pikhart H, Hertzman C, Rose R, Marmot M. 1998. Socioeconomic factors, perceived control and self-reported health in Russia. A cross-sectional survey. *Social Science and Medicine* 47(2):269-279.

Bogart LM, Catz SL, Kelly JA, Benotsch EG. 2001. Factors influencing physician's judgments of adherence and treatment decisions for patients with HIV disease. *Medical Decision Making* 21(1):28-36.

Bohlin G, Eliasson K, Hjemdahl P, Klein K, Fredrikson M, Frankenhaeuser M. 1986a. Personal control over work pace-circulaory, neuroendocrine and subjective responses in borderline hypertension. *Journal of Hypertension* 4:295-305.

Bohlin G, Eliasson K, Hjemdahl P, Klein K, Frankenhaeuser M. 1986b. Pace variation and control of work pace as related to cardiovascular, neuroendocrine, and subjective responses. *Biological Psychology* 23:247-263.

Bolen JC, Rhodes L, Powell-Griner EE, Bland SD, Holtzman D. 2000. State-specific prevalence of selected health behaviors, by race and ethnicity—Behavioral Risk Factor Surveillance System, 1997. *Morbidity and Mortality Weekly Report: Surveillance Summaries* 49 (SS-2):1-60.

Bond GE, Burr R, McCurry SM, Graves AB, Larson EB. 2001. Alcohol, aging, and cognitive performance in a cohort of Japanese Americans aged 65 and older: The Kame project. *International Psychogeriatrics* 13(2):207-223.

Bond Huie SA, Hummer RA, Rogers RG. 2002. Individual and contextual risks of death among race and ethnic groups in the United States. Paper presented at the annual meetings of the Population Association of America, Atlanta, May 9-11.

Bornstein MH, Cote LR. 2001. Mother-infant interaction and acculturation: I. Behavioural comparisons in Japanese American and South American families. *International Journal of Behavioural Development* 25:549-563.

Bosma H, Marmot MG, Hemingway H, Nicholson AC, Brunner E, Stansfeld SA. 1997. Low job control and risk of coronary heart disease in Whitehall II (prospective cohort) study. *British Medical Journal* 22;314(7080):558-565.

Bradshaw D, Norman R, Laubscher R, Schneider M, Mbananga N, Steyn K. 2004. An exploratory investigation into racial disparities in the health of older South Africans. In National Research Council, *Critical Perspectives on Racial and Ethnic Differences in Health in Later Life*. Anderson NA, Bulatao RA, Cohen B, eds. Committee on Population, Division of Behavioral and Social Sciences and Education. Washington, DC: The National Academies Press.

Braveman P, Cubbin C, Marchi K, Egerter S, Chavez G. 2001. Measuring socioeconomic status/position in studies of racial/ethnic disparities: Maternal and infant health. *Public Health Report* 116(5):449-463.

Breier A, Albus M, Pickar D, Zahn TP, Wolkovitz OM, Paul SM. 1987. Controllable and uncontrollable stress in humans: Alterations in mood and neuroendocrine and psychophysiological function. *American Journal of Psychiatry* 144(11):1419-1425.

Brown ER, Ojeda VD, Wyn R, Levan R. 2000. *Racial and Ethnic Disparities in Access to Health Insurance and Health Care*. Los Angeles, CA: UCLA Center for Health Policy Research and the Henry J. Kaiser Family Foundation.

Brunner E, Marmot M, Nanchahal K, Shipley M, Stansfeld S, Juneja M, Alberti K. 1997. Social inequality in coronary risk: Central obesity and the metabolic syndrome. Evidence from the Whitehall II study. *Diabetologia* 40(11):1341-1349.

Brunner EJ, Hemingway H, Walker BR, Page M, Clarke P, Juneja M, Shipley MJ, Kumari M, Andrew R, Seckl JR, Papadopoulos A, Checkley S, Rumley A, Lowe GD, Stansfeld SA, Marmot MG. 2002. Adrenocortical, autonomic, and inflammatory causes of the metabolic syndrome: Nested case-control study. *Circulation* 106(21):2659-2665.

Bullard RD. 1994. Urban infrastructure: Social environmental, and health risks to African Americans. Pp. 315-330 in *Handbook of Black American Health: The Mosaic of Conditions, Issues, Policies, and Prospects*. Livingston IL, ed. Westport, CT: Greenwood Publishing.

Burdette WJ. 1998. *Cancer: Etiology, Diagnosis and Treatment*. New York: McGraw-Hill.

Burke GL, Arnold AM, Bild DE, Cushman M, Fried LP, Newman A, Nunn C, Robbins J. 2001. Factors associated with healthy aging: The cardiovascular health study. *Journal of the American Geriatrics Society* 49(3):254-262.

Burnam MA, Hough RL, Karno M, Escobar JI, Telles CA. 1987. Acculturation and lifetime prevalence of psychiatric disorders among Mexican Americans in Los Angeles. *Journal of Health and Social Behavior* 28(1):89-102.

Burroughs VJ, Maxey RW, Levy RA. 2002. Racial and ethnic differences in response to medicines: Towards individualized pharmaceutical treatment. *Journal of the National Medical Association* 94(10, Suppl):1-26.

Byrd WM, Clayton LA. 2002. *An American Health Dilemma: Race, Medicine, and Health Care in the United States 1900-2000*, Vol. 2. New York: Routledge.

Calle EE, Thun MJ, Petrelli JM, Rodriguez C, Heath CW Jr. 1999. Body-mass index and mortality in a prospective cohort of U.S. adults. *New England Journal of Medicine* 341(15):1097-1105.

Carroll D, Davey Smith G, Shipley MJ, Steptoe A, Brunner EJ, Marmot MG. 2001. Blood pressure reactions to acute psychological stress and future blood pressure status: A 10-year follow-up of men in the Whitehall II study. *Psychosomatic Medicine* 63:737-743.

Casas YG, Schiller BC, DeSouza CA, Seals DR. 2001. Total and regional body composition across age in healthy Hispanic and white women of similar socioeconomic status. *American Journal of Clinical Nutrition* 73(1):13-18.

Case A, Paxson C, Lubotsky DH. 2002. Economic status and health in childhood: The origins of the gradient. *American Economic Review* 92(5):1308-1334.

Case RB, Moss AJ, Case N, McDermott M, Eberly S. 1992. Living alone after myocardial infarction. Impact on prognosis. *Journal of the American Medical Association* 267:515-519.

Casper RC. 1995. Nutrition and its relationship to aging. *Experimental Gerontology* 30(3/4):299-314.

Chaloupka F, Pacula LL. 1998. *An Examination of Gender and Race Differences in Youth Smoking Responsiveness to Price and Tobacco Control Policies*. NBER Working Paper No. 6541. Cambridge, MA: National Bureau of Economic Research.

Chaloupka FJ, Warner KE. 2000. Economics of smoking. In *Handbook of Health Economics*, Vol. 1B. Culyer AJ, Newhouse JP, eds. Amsterdam: North-Holland.

Chandra A, Skinner JS. 2004. Geography and racial health disparities. In National Research Council, *Critical Perspectives on Racial and Ethnic Differences in Health in Later Life*. Anderson NA, Bulatao RA, Cohen B, eds. Committee on Population, Division of Behavioral and Social Sciences and Education. Washington, DC: The National Academies Press.

Chandra RK, Singh G, Shridhara B. 1989. Effect of feeding whey hydrolysate, soy and conventional cow milk formulas on incidence of atopic disease in high risk infants. *Annals of Allergy* 63:102-106.

Christensen K, Vaupel JW, Holm NV, Yashin AI. 1995. Mortality among twins after age 6: Fetal origins hypothesis versus twin method. *British Medical Journal* 310(6977):432-436.

Chung H, Mahler JC, Kakuma T. 1995. Racial differences in treatment of psychiatric inpatients. *Psychiatric Services* 46(6):586-591.

Clark R. 2004. Significance of perceived racism: Toward understanding ethnic-group disparities in health, the later years. In National Research Council, *Critical Perspectives on Racial and Ethnic Differences in Health in Later Life*. Anderson NA, Bulatao RA, Cohen B, eds. Committee on Population, Division of Behavioral and Social Sciences and Education. Washington, DC: The National Academies Press.

Clark R, Anderson NB, Clark VR, Williams DR. 1999. Racism as a stressor for African Americans: A biopsychosocial model. *American Psychologist* 54(10):805-816.

Cleeland CS, Gonin R, Baez L, Loehrer P, Pandya KJ. 1997. Pain and treatment of pain in minority patients with cancer: The Eastern Cooperative Oncology Group Minority Outpatient Pain Study. *Annals of Internal Medicine* 127(9):813-816.

Coe C. 1999. Psychosocial factors and psychoneuroimmunology within a lifespan perspective. Pp. 201-219 in *Developmental Health and the Wealth of Nations*, Keating D, Hertzman C, eds. New York: Guilford Press.

Cohen S, Williamson GM. 1991. Stress and infectious disease in humans. *Psychological Bulletin* 109:5-24.

Cohen S, Tyrrell D, Smith A. 1991. Psychological stress and susceptibility to the common cold. *New England Journal of Medicine* 325:606-612.

Cohen S, Kessler R, Gordon L. 1998. *Measuring Stress: A Guide for Health and Social Scientists*. Oxford University Press.

Colantonio A, Kasl SV, Ostfeld AM, Berkman LF. 1993. Psychosocial predictors of stroke outcomes in an elderly population. *Journal of Gerontology* 48:S261-S268.

Coleman DL, Hummel KP. 1975. Symposium IV: Diabetic syndrome in animals. Influence of genetic background on the expression of mutations at the diabetes locus in the mouse. II. Studies on background modifiers. *Israel Journal of Medical Sciences* 11(7):708-713.

Collins KS, Tenney K, Hughes DL. 2002. *Quality of health care for African Americans: Findings from the Commonwealth Fund 2001 Health Care Quality Survey*. New York: The Commonwealth Fund.

Cooper RM, Zubek JP. 1958. Effects of enriched and restricted early environments on the learning ability of bright and dull rats. *Canadian Journal of Psychology* 12:159-164.

Cooper RS, David R. 1986. The biological concept of race and its application to public health and epidemiology. *Journal of Health and Politics, Policy and Law* 11:97-116.

Cooper RS, Steinhauer M, Schatzkin A, Miller W. 1981. Improved mortality among U.S. black, 1968-1978: The role of antiracist struggle. *International Journal of Health Services* 11:511-522.

Council on Ethical and Judicial Affairs. 1990. Black-white disparities in health care. *Journal of the American Medical Association* 263:2344-2355.

Crespo CJ, Smith E, Andersen RE, Carter-Pokras O, Ainsworth BE. 2000. Race/ethnicity, social class and their relation to physical inactivity during leisure time: Results from the Third National Health and Nutrition Examination Survey, 1988-1994. *American Journal of Preventive Medicine* 18(1):46-53.

Crimmins EM. 2001. Mortality and health in human life spans. *Experimental Gerontology* 36(4-6):885-897.

Crimmins EM, Hayward MD, Seeman T. 2004. Race/ethnicity, socioeconomic status and health. In National Research Council, *Critical Perspectives on Racial and Ethnic Differences in Health in Later Life*. Anderson NA, Bulatao RA, Cohen B, eds. Committee on Population, Division of Behavioral and Social Sciences and Education. Washington, DC: The National Academies Press.

Crow JF. 2002. Unequal by nature: A geneticist's perspective on human differences. *Dædalus: Journal of the American Academy of Arts and Sciences* (Winter):81-88.

Cunningham PJ. 1996. Healthcare utilization, expenditures, and insurance coverage for American Indians and Alaska Natives eligible for the Indian Health Service. Pp. 289-314 in National Research Council, *Changing Numbers, Changing Needs: American Indian Demography and Public Health*. Sandefur GD, Rindfuss RR, Cohen B, eds. Committee on Population, Commission on Behavioral and Social Sciences and Education. Washington, DC: National Academy Press.

Cutler DM. 2004. Behavioral health interventions: What works and why? In National Research Council, *Critical Perspectives on Racial and Ethnic Differences in Health in Later Life*. Anderson NA, Bulatao RA, Cohen B, eds. Committee on Population, Division of Behavioral and Social Sciences and Education. Washington, DC: The National Academies Press.

Cutler DM, Glaeser EL, Shapiro JM. 2003. *Why Have Americans Become More Obese?* NBER Working Paper No. 9446. Cambridge, MA: National Bureau of Economic Research.

Dalgard OS, Lund Haheim L. 1998. Psychosocial risk factors and mortality: A prospective study with special focus on social support, social participation, and locus of control in Norway. *Journal of Epidemiology and Community Health* 52(8):476-481.

Darnay AJ, ed. 1994. *Statistical Record of Older Americans.* Washington, DC: Gale Research Inc.

Davis JA, Smith TW. 1990. *General Social Surveys, 1972-1990 NORC Ed.* Chicago: National Opinion Research Center.

Davis MA, Neuhaus JM, Moritz DJ, Lein D, Barclay JD, Murphy SP. 1994. Health behaviors and survival among middle-aged and older men and women in the NHANES I Epidemiologic Follow-up Study. *Preventive Medicine* 23(3):369-376.

Dawson DA. 1998. Beyond black, white and Hispanic: Race, ethnic origin and drinking patterns in the United States. *Journal of Substance Abuse* 10(4):321-339.

Deaton A. 2002. Policy implications of the gradient of health and wealth. *Health Affairs* 21(2):13-30.

Deaton A, Paxson C. 2001. Mortality, education, income and income inequality among American cohorts. In *Themes in the Economics of Aging.* Wise DA, ed. Chicago: University of Chicago Press.

Decker S, Rapaport C. 2002. *Medicare and Disparities in Women's Health.* NBER Working Paper No. 8761, January. Cambridge, MA: National Bureau of Economic Research.

Desai M, Pratt LA, Lentzner H, Robinson KN. 2001. Trends in vision and hearing among older Americans. *Aging Trends,* No. 2. Hyattsville, MD: National Center for Health Statistics.

Dilworth-Anderson P, Gibson BE. 2002. The cultural influence of values, norms, meanings and perceptions in understanding dementia in ethnic minorities. *Alzheimer Disease and Associated Disorders* 16(Suppl. 2):S56-S63.

Doblhammer G. 2002. Differences in *Lifespan by Month of Birth for the United States: The Impact of Early Life Events and Conditions on Late Life Mortality.* MPIDR Working Paper 2002-19. Rostock, Germany: Max-Planck Institute for Demographic Research.

Dolk H, Vrijheid M, Armstrong B, Abramsky L, Bianchi F, Garne E, Nelen V, Robert E, Scott JE, Stone D, Tenconi R. 1998. Risk of congenital anomalies near hazardous-waste landfill sites in Europe: The EUROHAZCON study. *Lancet* 352(9126):423-427.

Dominitz JA, Samsa GP, Landsman P, Provenzale D. 1998. Race, treatment, and survival among colorectal carcinoma patients in an equal-access medical system. *Cancer* 82:2312-2320.

Doty MM, Ives BL. 2002. *Quality of Health Care for Hispanic Populations: Findings from The Commonwealth Fund 2001 Health Care Quality Survey.* New York: The Commonwealth Fund.

Dougal AL, Baum A. 2001. Stress, health, and illness. Pp. 321-337 in *Handbook of Health Psychology.* Baum A, Revenson T, Singer J, eds. Mahwah, NJ: Lawrence Erlbaum Associates.

Dufouil C, Ducimetiere P, Alperovitch A. 1997. Sex differences in the association between alcohol consumption and cognitive performance. *American Journal of Epidemiology* 146:405-412.

Eckardt MJ, File SE, Gessa GL, Grant KA, Guerri C, Hoffman PL, Kalant H, Koob GF, Li TK, Tabakoff B. 1998. Effects of moderate alcohol consumption on the central nervous system. *Alcoholism: Clinical and Experimental Research* 22(5):998-1040.

Economic Report of the President. 1998. Washington, DC: U.S. Government Printing Office.

Elias PK, Elias MF, D'Agostino RB, Silbershatz H, Wolf PA. 1999. Alcohol consumption and cognitive performance in the Framingham Heart Study. *American Journal of Epidemiology* 6:580-589.

Elo IT, Preston SH. 1992. Effects of early-life conditions on adult mortality: A review. *Population Index* 58(2):186-212.

Emmons KM. 2001. Behavioral and social science contributions to the health of adults in the United States. Pp. 254-321 in National Research Council, *Promoting Health: Intervention Strategies from Social and Behavioral Research.* Smedley BD, Syme SL, eds. Washington, DC: National Academy Press.

Erwin D, Spatz T, Stotts R, Hollenberg J. 1999. Increasing mammography practice by African American women. *Cancer Practice* 7(2):78-85.

Escarce JJ, Epstein KR, Colby DC, Schwartz JS. 1993. Racial differences in the elderly's use of medical procedures and diagnostic tests. *American Journal of Public Health* 83(7):948-954.

Espino DV, Burge SK, Moreno CA. 1991. The prevalence of selected chronic diseases among the Mexican-American elderly: Data from the 1982-1984 Hispanic Health and Nutrtion Examination Survey. *Journal of the American Board of Family Practice* 4:217-222.

Ettinger WH Jr, Burns R, Messier SP, Applegate W, Rejeski WJ, Morgan T, Shumaker S, Berry MJ, O'Toole M, Monu J, Craven T. 1997. A randomized trial comparing aerobic exercise and resistance exercise with a health education program in older adults with knee osteoarthritis. The Fitness Arthritis and Seniors Trial (FAST). *Journal of the American Medical Association* 277(1):25-31.

Evans GW, Kantrowitz E. 2002. Socioeconomic status and health: The potential role of environmental risk exposure. *Annual Review of Public Health* 23:303-331.

Evans GW, Saegert S. 2000. Residential crowding in the context of inner city poverty. Pp. 247-267 in *Theoretical Perspectives in Environment-Behavior Research.* Wapner S, Demick J, Yamamoto T, Minami H, Yamamoto CT, eds. New York: Kluwer Academic/ Plenum Publishers.

Ewbank D, Jones N. 2001. *Preliminary observations on the variations in the risk of death.* Paper presented at the annual meetings of the Population Association of America, Washington DC, March 29.

Exner DV, Dries DL, Domanski MJ, Cohn JN. 2001. Lesser response to angiotensin-converting-enzyme inhibitor therapy in black as compared with white patients with left ventricular dysfunction. *New England Journal of Medicine* 344:1351-1357.

Eyler AA, Whiteson RC, Donatelle RJ, King AC, White D, Sallis JF. 1999. Physical activity social support and middle- and older-aged minority women: Results from a US survey. *Social Science and Medicine* 49(6):781-789.

Faber DR, Krieg EJ. 2002. Unequal exposure to ecological hazards: Environmental injustices in the Commonwealth of Massachusetts. *Health Perspect* 110(Suppl 2):277-288.

Fabrigoule C, Letenneur L, Dartigues JF, Zarrouk M, Commenges D, Barberger-Gateau P. 1995. Social and leisure activities and risk of dementia: A prospective longitudinal study. *Journal of the American Geriatrics Society* 43:485-490.

Falkner B, Kushner H, Onesti G, Angelakos E. 1981. Cardiovascular characters in adolescents who develop essential hypertension. *Hypertension* 3:521-527.

Fall C, Hindmarsh P, Dennison E, Kellingray S, Barker D, Cooper C. 1998. Programming of growth hormone secretion and bone mineral density in elderly men: A hypothesis. *Journal of Clinical Endocrinology and Metabolism* 83(1):135-139.

Farley JH, Hines JF, Taylor RR, Carlson JW, Parker MF, Kost ER, Rogers SJ, Harrison TA, Macri CI, Parham GP. 2001. Equal care ensures equal survival for African-American women with cervical carcinoma. *Cancer* 91(4):869-873.

Feder J, Komisar HL, Niefeld M. 2001. The financing and organization of health care. Pp. 387-405 in *Handbook of Aging and the Social Sciences*, 5th ed. Binstock RH, George LK, eds. San Diego: Academic Press.

Federal Interagency Forum on Aging Related Statistics. 2000. *Older Americans 2000: Key Indicators of Well-Being*. Washington, DC.

Felitti VJ, Anda RF, Nordenberg D, Williamson DF, Spitz AM, Edwards V, Koss MP, Marks JS. 1998. Relationship of childhood abuse and household dysfunction to many of the leading causes of death in adults: The Adverse Childhood Experiences (ACE) study. *American Journal of Preventive Medicine* 14(4):245-258.

Fernando S. 1984. Racism as a cause of depression. *International Journal of Social Psychology* 30:41-49.

Finch BK, Hummer RA, Reindl M, Vega WA. 2002. Validity of self-rated health among Latino(a)s. *American Journal of Epidemiology* 155(8):755-759.

Finucane TE, Carrese JA. 1990. Racial bias in presentation of cases. *Journal of General Internal Medicine* 5(2):120-121.

Fix M, Struyk RJ, eds. 1993. *Clear and Convincing Evidence: Measurement of Discrimination in America*. Washington, DC: Urban Institute Press.

Forsdahl A. 1978. Living conditions in childhood and subsequent development of risk factors for arteriosclerotic heart disease. *Journal of Epidemiology and Community Health* 32:34-37.

Forsdahl A. 2002. Commentary: Childhood deprivation and adult mortality. *International Journal of Epidemiology* 31.

Fox AJ, Goldblatt PO, Jones DR. 1985. Social class mortality differentials: Artifact, selection or life circumstances? *Journal of Epidemiology and Community Health* 39(1):1-8.

Francis D, Diorio J, Liu D, Meaney MJ. 1999. Nongenomic transmission across generations of maternal behavior and stress responses in the rat. *Science* 286(5442):1155-1158.

Frankenhaeuser M, Johansson G. 1986. Stress at work: Psychobiological and psychosocial aspects. *International Review of Applied Psychology* 35:287-299.

Franzini L, Ribble JC, Keddie AM. 2001. Understanding the Hispanic paradox. *Ethnicity and Disease* 11(3):496-518.

Fratiglioni L, Wang HX, Ericsson K, Maytan M, Winblad B. 2000. Influence of social network on occurrence of dementia: A community-based longitudinal study. *Lancet* 355:1315-1319.

Galanis DJ, Joseph C, Masaki KH, Petrovitch H, Ross GW, White L. 2000. A longitudinal study of drinking and cognitive performance in elderly Japanese-American men: The Honolulu Asia Aging Study. *American Journal of Public Health* 90(8):1254-1259.

Gallant MP, Dorn GP. 2001. Gender and race differences in the predictors of daily health practices among older adults. *Health Education Research* 16(1):21-31.

Geiger J. 2003. *Unequal Treatment: Confronting Racial and Ethnic Disparities in Health Care*. Institute of Medicine. Smedley BD, Stith AY, Nelson AR, eds. Washington, DC: The National Academies Press.

Glass TA. 2000. Psychosocial interventions. Pp. 267-305 in *Social Epidemiology*. Berkman LF, Kawachi I, eds. New York: Oxford University Press.

Glass TA, Matchar DB, Belyea M, Feussner, JR. 1993. Impact of social support on outcome in first stroke. *Stroke* 24:64-70.

Glass TA, Mendes de Leon CF, Marottoli RA, Berkman LF. 1999. Population based study of social and productive activities as predictors of survival among elderly. *British Medical Journal* 319:478-483.

Glass TA, Dym B, Greenberg S, Rintell D, Roesch C, Berkman LF. 2000. Psychosocial intervention in stroke: The Families in Recovery from Stroke Trial (FIRST). *American Journal of Orthopsychiatry* 70:169-181.

Goldberg MS, Siemiatyck J, DeWar R. 1999. Risks of developing cancer relative to living near a municipal solid waste landfill site in Montreal, Quebec, Canada. *Archives of Environmental Health* 54(4):291-296.

Goldman DP, Smith JP. 2002. Can patient self-management help explain the SES health gradient? *Proceedings of the National Academy of Sciences* 99(16):10929-10934.

Goldman N. 2001. Social inequalities in health: Disentangling the underlying mechanisms. In *Population Health and Aging: Strengthening the Dialogue Between Epidemiology and Demography.* Weinstein M, Hermalin AI, Stoto MA, eds. Demography and Epidemiology: Frontiers in Population Health and Aging. New York: New York Academy of Sciences.

Gornick M. 2000. *Vulnerable Populations and Medicare Services: Why Do Disparities Exist?* New York: Century Foundation Press.

Gostin LO. 2001. Legal and public policy interventions to advance the populations health. Pp. 390-416 in National Research Council, *Promoting Health: Intervention Strategies from Social and Behavioral Research.* Smedley BD, Syme SL, eds. Washington, DC: National Academy Press.

Gott CM. 2001. Sexual activity and risk-taking in later life. *Health and Social Care in the Community* 9(2):72-78.

Grabowski DC, Ellis JE. 2001. High body mass index does not predict mortality in older people: Analysis of the Longitudinal Study of Aging. *Journal of the American Geriatrics Society* 49(7):968-979.

Greeley AM. 1989. *Religious Change in America.* Cambridge, MA: Harvard University Press.

Grossman, DC. 2003. Measuring disparity among American Indians and Alaska Natives: Who's counting whom? *Medical Care* 41(5):579-581.

Gruber J, Kosygi B. 2002. *A Theory of Government Regulation of Addictive Bads: Optimal Tax Levels and Tax Incidence for Cigarette Excise Taxation.* NBER Working Paper No. 8777, February.

Gump BB, Matthews KA, Räikkönen K. 1999. Modeling relationships among socioeconomic status, hostility, cardiovascular reactivity, and left ventricular mass in African American and white children. *Health Psychology* 18(2):140-150.

Guyll M, Matthews KA, Bromberger JT. 2001. Discrimination and unfair treatment: Relationship to cardiovascular reactivity among African American and European American women. *Health Psychology* 20(5):315-325.

Gwatkin DR. 2000. Health inequalities and the health of the poor: What do we know? What can we do? *Bulletin of the World Health Organization* 78(1):3-18.

Hack M, Flannery DJ, Schluchter M, Carter L, Borawski E, Klein N. 2002. Outcomes in young adulthood for very-low-birth-weight infants. *New England Journal of Medicine* 346(3):149-157.

Hahn R, Vesely S, Chang M-H. 2000. Health risk aversion, health risk affinity, and socioeconomic position in the USA: The demographics of multiple risk. *Health, Risk and Society* 2(3):295-314.

Hallback M. 1975. Interaction between central neurogenic mechanisms and changes in cardiovascular design in primary hypertension: Experimental studies in spontaneously hypertensive rats. *Acta Physiologica Scandinavica* 424(Suppl):1-59.

Harrell JP, Merritt MM, Kalu J. 1998. Racism, stress, and disease. Pp. 247-280 in *African American Mental Health.* Jones RL, ed. Hampton, VA: Cobb and Henry Publishers.

Harrell JP, Hall S, Talliaferro J. 2003. Physiological responses to racism and discrimination: An assessment of the evidence. *American Journal of Public Health* 93(2):243-248.

Harris DR, Sim JJ. 2002. Who is multiracial? Assessing the complexity of lived race. *American Sociological Review* 67(4):614-628.

Hartl DL, Clark AG. 1997. *Principles of Population Genetics.* 3rd ed. Sunderland, MA: Sinauer Associates.

Hayward MD, Gorman BK. 2002. *The Long Arm of Childhood: The Influence of Early Life Social Conditions on Men's Mortality.* University Park, PA: Population Research Institute.

Hayward MD, Heron M. 1999. Racial inequality in active life expectancy among adult Americans. *Demography* 36:77-91.

Hayward MD, Crimmins EM, Miles TP, Yang Y. 2000. The significance of socioeconomic status in explaining the racial gap in chronic health conditions. *American Sociological Review* 65:910-930.

He W. 2002. The older foreign-born population in the United States: 2000. *Current Population Reports,* Series P23-211. Washington, DC: U.S. Government Printing Office.

Hebb JH, Fitzgerald D, Fan W. 2003. Healthcare disparities in disadvantaged Medicare beneficiaries: A national project overview. *Journal of Health and Human Services Administration* 25(3).

Henselman LW, Henderson D, Shadoan J, Subramaniam M, Saunders S, Ohlin D. 1995. Effects of noise exposure, race, and years of service on hearing in U.S. Army soldiers. *Ear and Hearing* 16(4):382-391.

Herholz H, Goff DC, Ramsey DJ, Chan FA, Ortiz C, Labarthe DR, Nichaman MZ. 1996. Women and Mexican Americans receive fewer cardiovascular drugs following myocardial infarction than men and non-Hispanic whites: The Corpus Christi Heart project, 1988-1990. *Journal of Clinical Epidemiology* 49(3):279-287.

Heron WT. 1935. The inheritance of maze learning ability in rats. *Journal of Comparative Psychology* 19:77-89.

Hertzman C. 2004. The life course contribution to ethnic disparities in health. In National Research Council, *Critical Perspectives on Racial and Ethnic Differences in Health in Later Life.* Anderson NA, Bulatao RA, Cohen B, eds. Committee on Population, Division of Behavioral and Social Sciences and Education. Washington, DC: The National Academies Press.

Hertzman C, McLean S, Kohen D, Dunn J, Evans T. 2002. Early development in Vancouver: Report of the Community Asset Mapping Project. Available: http:// www.earlylearning.ucb.ca [Accessed December 2002].

Hill ME, Preston SH, Rosenwaike I. 2000. Age reporting among white Americans aged 85+: Results of a record linkage study. *Demography* 37:175-186.

Himes CL, Reynolds SL. 2002. *Trends in obesity and educational status: The risk of negative health outcomes for future cohorts of older adults.* Paper presented at the annual meeting of the Population Association of America, Atlanta, May 9-11.

Hitt R, Young-Xu Y, Silver M, Perls T. 1999. Centenarians: The older you get, the healthier you have been. *Lancet* 354(9179):652.

Hjemdahl P. 2002. Stress and the metabolic syndrome: An interesting but enigmatic association. *Circulation* 106:2634-2636.

Hoffman AA, Parsons PA. 1991. *Evolutionary Genetics and Environmental Stress.* Oxford, UK: Oxford University Press.

Hogue CJR, Hargraves MA. 1993. Class, race, and infant mortality in the United States. (Commentary). *American Journal of Public Health* 83(1):9-12.

Hogue CJ, Hargraves MA, Collins KS, eds. 2000. *Minority Health in America: Findings and Policy Implications from the Commonwealth Fund Minority Health Survey.* Baltimore: Johns Hopkins University Press.

House JS, Williams DR. 2000. Understanding and reducing socioeconomic and racial/ethnic disparities in health. Pp. 81-124 in National Research Council, *Promoting Health: Intervention Strategies from Social and Behavioral Research*. Smedley BD, Syme SL, eds. Washington, DC: National Academy Press.

House JS, Lepkowski JM, Kinney AM, Mero RP, Kessler RC, Herzog AR. 1994. The social stratification of aging and health. *Journal of Health and Social Behavior* 35:213-234.

Hoyert DL, Kung H. 1997. Asian or Pacific Islander mortality, selected states, 1992. *Monthly Vital Statistics Report* 46(1,Suppl).

Hoyert DL, Arias E, Smith BL, Murphy SL, Kochanek KD. 2001. Deaths: Final data for 1999. *National Vital Statistics Reports* 49(8). National Center for Health Statistics.

Hudson RB. 2002. Workers of color and pathways to retirement. In *Public Policy and Aging Report, Spring 2002*. Hudson RB, ed. Washington, DC: Gerontological Society of America.

Hughes DL. 2002. *Quality of Health Care for Asian Americans: Findings from the Commonwealth Fund 2001 Health Care Quality Survey*. New York: The Commonwealth Fund.

Hummer RA, Rogers RG, Eberstein IW. 1998. Sociodemographic differentials in adult mortality: A review of analytic approaches. *Population and Development Review* 24(3):553-578.

Hummer RA, Rogers RG, Nam CB, Ellison CG. 1999. Religious involvement and U.S. adult mortality. *Demography* 36:273-285.

Hummer R, Benjamins MR, Rogers RG. 2004. Racial and ethnic disparities in health and mortality among the U.S. elderly population. In National Research Council, *Critical Perspectives on Racial and Ethnic Differences in Health in Later Life*. Committee on Population, Anderson NA, Bulatao RA, Cohen B, eds. Division of Behavioral and Social Sciences and Education. Washington, DC: The National Academies Press.

Idler EL, Kasl SV. 1997. Religion among disabled and nondisabled persons II: Attendance at religious services as a predictor of the course of disability. *Journals of Gerontology Series B, Psychological Sciences and Social Sciences* 52(6):306-316.

Ignatiev N. 1995. *How the Irish Became White*. New York: Routledge.

Independent Inquiry into Inequalities in Health: Report. 1998. London: Stationery Office.

Indian Health Service. 1999. *Trends in Indian Health, 1998-99*. Available: http://www.ihs.gov/PublicInfo/Publications/trends98/trends98.asp [Accessed March 2003].

Institute of Medicine. 2003. *Unequal Treatment: Confronting Racial and Ethnic Disparities in Health Care*. Smedley BD, Stith AY, Nelson AR, eds. Committee on Understanding and Eliminating Racial and Ethnic Disparities in Health Care, Board on Health Sciences Policy. Washington, DC: The National Academies Press.

Jackson JS, Ramon C. 2002. "A mind is a terrible thing to lose": Health and mental health disparities among ethnic and racial minorities. *Current Directions in Psychological Science*.

Jackson JS, White TB, Williams DR, Torres M, Sellers SL, White K. 1996. Racism and the physical and mental health status of African Americans: A thirteen-year national panel study. *Ethnicity and Disease* 6(1,2):132-147.

Jackson JS, Williams DR, Torres M. 2003. Perceptions of discrimination: The stress process and physical and psychological health. In *Social Stressors, Personal and Social Resources, and Their Mental Health Consequences*. Maney A, ed. Washington, DC: National Institute for Mental Health.

James SA. 1999. Primordial prevention of cardiovascular disease among African-Americans: a social epidemiological perspective. *Preventive Medicine* 29(6 Pt 2):S84-S89.

James SA, LaCroix AZ, Kleinbaum DG, Strogatz DS. 1984. John Henryism and blood pressure differences among black men II: The role of occupational stressors. *Journal of Behavioral Medicine* 7:259-275.

Jasso G, Massey DS, Rosenzweig MR, Smith JP. 2000. The New Immigrant Survey Pilot (NIS-P): Overview and new findings about U.S. legal immigrants at admission. *Demography* 37:127-138.

Jasso G, Massey DS, Rosenzweig MR, Smith JP. 2004. Immigrant health—Selectivity and acculturation. In National Research Council, *Critical Perspectives on Racial and Ethnic Differences in Health in Later Life*. Anderson NA, Bulatao RA, Cohen B, eds. Committee on Population, Division of Behavioral and Social Sciences and Education. Washington, DC: The National Academies Press.

Jencks SF, Cuerdon T, Bower DR, Fleming B, Houck PM, Kussmaul AE, Nilasen DS, Ordin DL, Arday DR. 2000. Quality of medical care delivered to Medicare beneficiaries: A profile at state and national levels. *Journal of the American Medical Association* 284(13):1670-1676.

Jerger J, Jerger S, Pepe P, Miller R. 1986. Race difference in susceptibility to noise-induced hearing loss. *American Journal of Otology* 7(6):425-429.

Jiang W, Babyak M, Krantz DS, Waugh RA, Coleman E, Hanson MM, Frid DJ, McNulty S, Morris JJ, O'Connor CM, Blumenthal JA. 1996. Mental stress-induced myocardial ischemia and cardiac events. *Journal of the American Medical Association* 275:1651-1656.

Jones J. 2001. Ethnicity may affect alternative, complementary therapy choices. *Journal of the National Cancer Institute* 93(20):1522-1523.

Jones JM. 1997. *Prejudice and Racism*. 2nd ed. New York: McGraw-Hill.

Kagawa-Singer M, Hikoyeda N, Tanjasiri SP. 1997. Aging, chronic conditions, and physical disabilities in Asian and Pacific Islander Americans. In *Minorities, Aging and Health*. Markides KS, Miranda MR, eds. Thousand Oaks, CA: Sage Publications.

Kahn KL, Pearson ML, Harrison ER, Desmond KA, Rogers WH, Rubenstein LV, Brook RH, Keeler EB. 1994. Health care for black and poor hospitalized Medicare patients. *Journal of the American Medical Association* 271(15):1169-1174.

Kales HC, Blow FC, Bingham CR, Roberts JC, Copeland LA, Mellow AM. 2000. Race, psychiatric diagnosis, and mental health care utilization in older patients. *American Journal of Geriatric Psychiatry* 8(4):301-309.

Kalmijn S, van Boxtel MP, Verschuren MW, Jolles J, Launer LJ. 2002. Cigarette smoking and alcohol consumption in relation to cognitive performance in middle age. *American Journal of Epidemiology* 156(10):936-944.

Kaplan GA, Everson SA, Lynch JW. 2000. The contribution of social and behavioral research to an understanding of the distribution of disease: A multilevel approach. Pp. 37-80 in National Research Council, *Promoting Health: Intervention Strategies From Social and Behavioral Research*. Smedley BD, Syme SL, eds. Washington, DC: National Academy Press.

Kaplan R, Sallis J, Patterson TL. 1993. *Health and Human Behavior*. New York: McGraw-Hill.

Karasek RA, Theorell T, Schwartz JE, Schnall PL, Pieper CF, Michela JL. 1988. Job characteristics in relation to the prevalence of myocardial infarction in the US Health Examination Survey (HES) and the Health and Nutrition Survey Examination Survey (HANES). *American Journal of Public Health* 78(8):910-918.

Karter AJ, Ferrara A, Liu JY, Moffet HH, Ackerson LM, Selby JV. 2002. Ethnic disparities in diabetic complications in an insured population. *Journal of the American Medical Association* 287:2519-2527.

Kasim-Karakas SF. 2000. Ethnic differences in the insulin resistance syndrome. *American Journal of Clinical Nutrition* 71(3):670-671.

Kaufman JS, Cooper RS, McGee DL. 1997. Socioeconomic status and health in black and whites: The problem of residual confounding and the resiliency of race. *Epidemiology* 8(6):621-628.

Keeler GJ, Dvonch JT, Fuyuen Y, Parker EA, Israel BA, Marsik FJ, Morishita M, Barres JA, Robins TG, Brakefield-Caldwell W, Sam M. 2002. Assessment of personal and community-level exposures to particulate matter among children with asthmas in Detroit, Michigan, as part of Community Action Against Asthma (CAAA). *Environmental Health Perspectives* 110:173-181.

Kessler RC, Neighbors HW. 1986. A new perspective on the relationships among race, social class, and psychological distress. *Journal of Health and Social Behavior* 27(2):107-115.

Kiecolt-Glaser JK. 1999. Stress, personal relationships, and immune function: Health implications. *Brain, Behavior, and Immunity* 13:61-72.

Kiecolt-Glaser JK, Glaser R. 1995. Psychoneuroimmunology and health consequences: Data and shared mechanisms. *Psychosomatic Medicine.*

Kiecolt-Glaser JK, Glaser R, Dyer C, Shuttleworth E, Ogrocki P, Speicher CE. 1987. Chronic stress and immunity in family caregivers of Alzheimer's disease victims. *Psychosomatic Medicine* 49:523-535.

Kiecolt-Glaser JK, Malarkey W, Cacioppo JT, Glaser R. 1994. Stressful personal relationships: Endocrine and immune function. Pp. 321-339 in *Handbook of Human Stress and Immunity*. Glaser R, Kiecolt-Glaser JK, eds. San Diego, CA: Academic Press.

Kiely DK, Simon SE, Jones RN, Morris JN. 2000. The protective effect of social engagement on mortality in long-term care. *Journal of the American Geriatrics Society* 48, 1367-1372.

Kim Y. 2002. The role of cognitive control in mediating the effect of stressful circumstances among Korean immigrants. *Health & Social Work* 27(1):36-46.

Kington RS, Smith JP. 1997. Socioeconomic and race and ethnic differences in functional status associated with chronic disease. *American Journal of Public Health* 87:805-810.

Kington, RS, Nickens HW. 2001. Racial and ethnic differences in health: Recent trends, current patterns, future directions. Pp. 253-310 in National Research Council, *America Becoming: Racial Trends and Their Consequences*, Vol. 2. Smelser N, Wilson WJ, Mitchell F, eds. Washington, DC: National Academy Press.

Klinenberg E. 2002. *Heat Wave: A Social Autopsy of Disaster in Chicago.* Chicago: University of Chicago Press.

Knowler WC, Barrett-Connor E, Fowler SE, Hamman RF, Lachin JM, Walker EA, Nathan DM. 2002. Diabetes Prevention Program Research Group. Reduction in the incidence of type 2 diabetes with lifestyle intervention or metformin. *New England Journal of Medicine* 346(6):393-403.

Koenig HG, George LK, Siegler IC. 1998. The use of religion and other emotion-related coping strategies among older adults. *Gerontologist* 18:303-310.

Koenig HG, Hays JC, Larson DB, George LK, Cohen HJ, McCullough ME, Meador KG, Blazer DG. 1999. Does religious attendance prolong survival? A six-year follow-up study of 3,968 older adults. *Journal of Gerontology Series A, Biological Sciences and Medical Sciences* 54(7):370-376.

Korenbrot CC, Ehlers S, Crouch JA. 2003. Disparities in hospitalizations of rural American Indians. *Medical Care* 41(5):626-636.

Kramarow E, Lentzner H, Rooks R, Weeks J, Saydah S. 1999. *Health, United States, 1999: Health and Aging Chartbook.* Hyattsville, MD: National Center for Health Statistics.

Krieger N. 1999. Embodying inequality: A review of concepts, measures, and methods for studying health consequences of discrimination. *International Journal of Health Services* 29(2):295-352.

Kubzansky LD, Berkman LF, Glass TA, Seeman TE. 1998. Is educational attainment associated with shared determinants of health in the elderly? Findings from the MacArthur Studies of Successful Aging. *Psychosomatic Medicine* 60(5):578-585.

Kubzansky L, Kawachi I, Sparrow D. 1999. Socioeconomic status, hostility, and risk factor clustering in the Normative Aging Study: Any help from the concept of allostatic load? *Annals of Behavioral Medicine* 21:330-338.

Kubzansky L, Berkman L, Seeman T. 2000. Social conditions and distress in elderly person: Findings from the MacArthur Studies of Successful Aging. *Journals of Gerontology, Series B: Psychological Sciences and Social Sciences* 55B(4):P238-P246.

Kuh D, Davey-Smith G. 1997. The life course and adult chronic disease: An historical perspective with particular reference to coronary heart disease. In *A Life Course Approach to Chronic Disease Epidemiology*. Kuh D, Ben-Shlomo B, eds. New York: Oxford University Press.

Kumanyika S. 1987. Obesity in black women. *Epidemiologic Reviews* 9:31-50.

Kuo WH. 1984. The prevalence of depression among Asian Americans. *Journal of Nervous and Mental Disease* 172:449-457.

Kuo WH, Porter K. 1998. Health status of Asian Americans: United States, 1992-94. *Advance Data from Vital Health Statistics*, No. 298. Hyattsville, MD: National Center for Health Statistics.

Laaksonen DE, Lakka HM, Niskanen LK, Kaplan GA, Salonen JT, Lakka TA. 2002. Metabolic syndrome and development of diabetes mellitus: Application and validation of recently suggested definitions of the metabolic syndrome in a prospective cohort study. *American Journal of Epidemiology* 156(11):1070-1077.

Lakka HM, Laaksonen DE, Lakka TA, Niskanen LK, Kumpusalo E, Tuomilehto J, Salonen JT. 2002. The metabolic syndrome and total and cardiovascular disease mortality in middle-aged men. *Journal of the American Medical Association* 288(21):2709-2716.

Landrine H, Klonoff EA. 1996. The schedule of racist events: A measure of racial discrimination and a study of its negative physical and mental health consequences. *Journal of Black Psychology* 22(2):144-168.

Langer E, Rodin J. 1976. The effects of choice and enhanced personal responsibility for the aged: A field experiment in an institutional setting. *Journal of Personality and Social Psychology* 34:191-198.

Lantz PM, Lynch JW, House JS, Lepkowski JM, Mero RP, Musick MA, Williams DR. 2001. Socioeconomic disparities in health change in a longitudinal study of US adults: The role of health-risk behaviors. *Social Science and Medicine* 53(1):29-40.

Lauderdale DS, Kestenbaum B. 2002. Mortality rates of elderly Asian American populations based on Medicare and Social Security data. *Demography* 39:529-540.

Launer LJ, Harris T, Rumpel C, Madans J. 1994. Body mass index, weight change and risk of mobility disability in middle aged and older women. *Journal of the American Medical Association* 271:1093-1098.

LaVeist TA, Wallace JM Jr. 2000. Health risk and inequitable distribution of liquor stores in African American neighborhoods. *Social Science and Medicine* 51:613-617.

LaVeist TA, Nickerson KJ, Bowie JV. 2000. Attitudes about racism, medical mistrust, and satisfaction with care among African American and white cardiac patients. *Medical Care Research and Review* 57 (Suppl 1):146-161.

Leon DA. 1995. Adult height and mortality in London: Early life, socioeconomic confounding, or shrinkage? *Journal of Epidemiology and Community Health* 49:5-9.

Levinson D, Ember M, eds. 1997. *American Immigrant Cultures: Builders of a Nation*. 2 vols. New York: Simon and Schuster Macmillan.

Liao Y, Cooper RS, Cao G, Durazo-Arvizu R, Kaufman JS, Luke A, McGee DL. 1998. Mortality patterns among adult Hispanics: Findings from the NHIS, 1986-1990. *American Journal of Public Health* 88:227-232.

Lieberson S, Waters MC. 1993. The ethnic responses of whites: What causes their instability, simplification, and inconsistency? *Social Forces* 72:421-450.

Light K, Dolan C, Davis M, Sherwood A. 1992. Cardiovascular responses to an active coping challenge as predictors of blood pressure patterns 10-15 years later. *Psychosomatic Medicine* 54:217-230.

Lillie-Blanton M, Brodie M, Rowland D, Altman D, McIntosh M. 2000. Race, ethnicity, and the health care system: Public perceptions and experiences. *Medical Care Research and Review* 57 (Suppl 1):218-235.

Lobel M, Dunkel-Schetter C, Scrimshaw S. 1992. Prenatal maternal stress and prematurity: A prospective study of socioeconomically disadvantaged women. *Health Psychology* 11(1):32-40.

Loera J, Black SA, Espino DV, Goodwin JS. 2001. The use of herbal medicines by older Mexican Americans. *Journals of Gerontology Series A: Biological Sciences and Medical Sciences* 56(11):M714-M718.

Lovallo WR, Wilson MF. 1992. A biobehavioral model of hypertension development. Pp. 265-280 in *Individual Differences in Cardiovascular Responses to Stress*. Turner JR, Sherwood A, Light KC, eds. New York: Plenum Press.

Lovejoy JC, de la Bretonne JA, Klemperer M, Tulley R. 1996. Abdominal fat distribution and metabolic risk factors: Effects of race. *Metabolism* 45:1119-1124.

Lowe RA, Chhaya S, Nasci K, Gavin LJ, Shaw K, Zwanger ML, Zeccardi JA, Dalsey WC, Abbuhl SB, Feldman H, Berlin JA. 2001. Effect of ethnicity on denial of authorization for emergency department care by managed care gatekeepers. *Academic Emergency Medicine* 8(3):259-266.

Lucas A. 1991. Programming by early nutrition in man. Pp. 38-55 in *The Childhood Environment and Adult Disease*, Bock GR, Whelen J, eds. Chichester: John Wiley.

Lucas A. 1994. Role of nutritional programming in determining adult morbidity. *Archives of Disease in Childhood* 71:288-290.

Lucas A, Fewtrell MS, Cole TJ. 1999. Fetal origins of adult disease—The hypothesis revisited. *British Medical Journal* 319:245-249.

Lundberg O. 1991. Childhood living conditions, health status, and social mobility. *European Sociological Review* 7(2):149-162.

Lurie N, Ward NB, Shapiro MF, Brook RH. 1984. Termination from Medi-Cal—Does it affect health? *New England Journal of Medicine* 311:480-484.

Mandinger M. 1985. Health service funding cuts and the declining health of the poor. *New England Journal of Medicine* 313:44-47.

Manly JJ, Mayeux R. 2004. Ethnic differences in dementia and Alzheimer's disease. In National Research Council, *Critical Perspectives on Racial and Ethnic Differences in Health in Later Life*. Anderson NA, Bulatao RA, Cohen B, eds. Committee on Population, Division of Behavioral and Social Sciences and Education. Washington, DC: The National Academies Press.

Mann B, Sherman L, Clayton C, Johnson R, Keates J, Kasenge R, Streeter K, Goldberg L, Nieman L. 2000. Screening to the converted: An educational intervention in African American churches. *Journal of Cancer Education* 15(1):46-50.

Manton K, Stallard E. 1984. *Recent Trends in Mortality Analysis*. New York: Academic Press.

Manton KG, Stallard E. 1997. Health and disability differences among racial and ethnic groups. Pp. 43-105 in National Research Council, *Racial and Ethnic Differences in the Health of Older Americans*. Committee on Population, Martin LG, Soldo BJ, eds. Commission on Behavioral and Social Sciences and Education. Washington, DC: National Academy Press.

Manuck S, Kasprowicz A, Muldoon M. 1990. Behaviorally-evoked cardiovascular reactivity and hypertension: Conceptual issues and potential associations. *Annals of Behavioral Medicine* 12:17-29.

Manuck SB, Marsland AL, Kaplan JR, Williams JK. 1995.The pathogenicity of behavior and its neuroendocrine mediation: An example from coronary artery disease. *Psychosomatic Medicine* 57(3):275-283.

Markides KS, Black S. 1996. Race, ethnicity, and aging: The impact of inequality. In *Handbook of Aging and the Social Sciences*. Binstock RH, George LK, eds. New York: Academic Press.

Marmot M. 2000. Multilevel approaches to understanding social determinants. Pp. 349-367 in *Social Epidemiology*. Berkman LF, Kawachi I, eds. Oxford, U.K.: Oxford University Press.

Marmot MG, Bosma H, Hemingway H, Brunner E, Stansfeld S. 1997a. Contribution of job control and other risk factors to social variations in coronary heart disease incidence. *Lancet* 350(9073):235-239.

Marmot M, Ryff C, Bumpass L, Shipley M, Marks N. 1997b. Social inequalities in health: Next question and converging evidence. *Social Science and Medicine* 44:901-910.

Martikainen P, Valkonen T. 1996. Mortality after death of spouse in relation to duration of bereavement in Finland. *Journal of Epidemiology and Community Health* 50(3):264-268.

Massey DS, Denton NA. 1993. *American Apartheid: Segregation and the Making of the Underclass*. Cambridge, MA: Harvard University Press.

Matthews K, Weiss S, Detre T. 1986. *Handbook of Stress, Reactivity, and Cardiovascular Disease*. New York: John Wiley and Sons.

Maxwell NL. 1994. The effect on black-white wage differences in the quantity and quality of education. *Industrial Labor Review* 47:249-264.

Mayberry RM, Mili F, Ofili E. 2000. Racial and ethnic differences in access to medical care. *Medical Care Research Review* 57(Suppl 1):108-145.

McAuley E. 1993. Self-efficacy, physical activity, and aging. Pp. 187-206 in *Activity and Aging: Staying Involved in Later Life*. Kelly JR, ed. Newbury Park: Sage Publications.

McBean AM, Gornick M. 1994. Differences by race in the rates of procedures performed in hospitals for Medicare beneficiaries. *Health Care Financing Review* 15(4):77-90.

McCarthy JD, Yancey WL. 1971. Uncle Tom and Mr. Charlie: Metaphysical pathos in the study of racism and personal disorganization. *American Journal of Sociology* 76:648-672.

McEwen B. 1998. Stress, adaptation, and disease. Allostasis and allostatic load. *Annals of New York Academy of Sciences* 840:33-44.

McEwen BS, Stellar E. 1993. Stress and the individual: Mechanisms leading to disease. *Archives of Internal Medicine* 153(18):2093-2101.

McGinnis JM, Foege WH. 1993. Actual causes of death in the United States. *Journal of the American Medical Association* 270(18):2207-2212.

McMahon A, Kvetnansky R, Fukuhara K, Weise WK, Kopin IJ, Sabban EL. 1992. Regulation of tyrosine hydroxylase and dopamine B-hydroxylase mRNA levels in rat adrenals by a single and repeated immobilization stress. *Journal of Neurochemistry* 58:2124-2130.

McNabb W, Quinn M, Kerver J, Cook S, Karrison T. 1997. The PATHWAYS church-based weight loss program for urban African-American women at risk for diabetes. *Diabetes Care* 20(10):1518-1523.

McNeilly MD, Anderson NB, Armstead CA, Clark R, Corbett M, Robinson EL, Pieper CF, Lepisto EM. 1996. A perceived racism scale: A multidimensional assessment of the experience of white racism among African Americans. *Ethnicity and Disease* 6(1,2):154-166.

Mendes de Leon C, Glass TA. 2004. The role of social networks and personal resources in ethnic disparities in aging health. In National Research Council, *Critical Perspectives on Racial and Ethnic Differences in Health in Later Life.* Anderson NA, Bulatao RA, Cohen B, eds. Committee on Population, Division of Behavioral and Social Sciences and Education. Washington, DC: The National Academies Press.

Mendes de Leon CF, Seeman TE, Baker DI, Richardson ED, Tinetti ME. 1996. Self-efficacy, physical decline, and change in functioning in community-living elders: A prospective study. *Journals of Gerontology: Social Sciences* 51:S183-S190.

Mendes de Leon CF, Glass TA, Beckett LA, Seeman TE, Evans DA, Berkman LF. 1999. Social networks and disability transitions across eight intervals of yearly data in the New Haven EPESE. *Journals of Gerontology Series B, Psychological Sciences and Social Sciences* 54:162-172.

Mendes de Leon CF, Gold DT, Glass TA, Kaplan L, George LK. 2001. Disability as a function of social networks and support in elderly African Americans and whites: The Duke EPESE 1986-1992. *Journals of Gerontology Series B, Psychological Sciences and Social Sciences* 56:S179-S190.

Menkes MS, Matthews KA, Krantz DS, Lundberg U, Mead LA, Qaqish B, Liang KY, Thomas CB, Pearson TA. 1989. Cardiovascular reactivity as to the cold pressor test as a predictor of hypertension. *Hypertension* 14(5):524-530.

Meyers S, Darity WA. 2000. Income and wealth. In *New Directions: African Americans in a Diversifying Nation.* Jackson JS, ed. Washington, DC: National Policy Association.

Miller B, Kolonel L, Bernstein L, Young J Jr, Swanson G, West D, Key D, Liff J, Glover C, Alexander G, et al., eds. 1996. *Racial/Ethnic Patterns of Cancer in the United States 1988-1992.* NIH Pub. No. 96-4101. Bethesda, MD.: National Cancer Institute.

Mirowsky J, Ross CE. 1990. Control or defense? Depression and the sense of control over good and bad outcomes. *Journal of Health and Social Behavior* 31(1):71-86.

Moffitt RA. 2003. *Causal and non-causal research in population: An economist's perspective.* Paper presented at the annual meeting of the Population Association of America, May 1-3, Minneapolis, MN.

Mohai P, Bryant B. 1992. Environmental racism: Reviewing the evidence. Pp. 163-176 in *Race and the Incidence of Environmental Hazards: A Time for Discourse.* Bryant B, Mohai P, eds. Boulder, CO: Westview Press.

Mohai P, Bryant B. 1998. Is there a race effect on concern for environmental quality? *Public Opinion Quarterly* 62(4):475-505.

Montague A. 1942. *Man's Most Dangerous Myth: The Fallacy of Race.* New York: Columbia University Press.

Moore RD, Stanton D, Gopalan R, Chaisson RE. 1994. Racial differences in the use of drug therapy for HIV disease in an urban community. *New England Journal of Medicine* 330(11):763-768.

Moore SE, Cole TJ, Poskitt EM, Sonko BJ, Whitehead RG, McGregor IA, Prentice AM. 1997. Season of birth predicts mortality in rural Gambia. *Nature* 388(6641):434.

Morenoff JD, Lynch J. 2004. What makes a place healthy? Neighborhood influences on racial/ethnic disparities in health over the life course. In National Research Council, *Critical Perspectives on Racial and Ethnic Differences in Health in Later Life.* Anderson NA, Bulatao RA, Cohen B, eds. Committee on Population, Division of Behavioral and Social Sciences and Education. Washington, DC: The National Academies Press.

Morrison RS, Wallenstein S, Natale DK, Senzel RS, Huang L-L. 2000. "We don't carry that"—Failure of pharmacies in predominantly nonwhite neighborhoods to stock opiod analgesics. *New England Journal of Medicine* 342:1023-1026.

Mukamel DB, Murthy AS, Weimer DL. 2000. Racial differences in access to high-quality cardiac surgeons. *American Journal of Public Health* 90:1774-1777.

Multiple Risk Factor Intervention Trial Research Group. 1982. Multiple Risk Factor Intervention Trial: Risk factor changes and mortality results. *Journal of the American Medical Association* 248(12):1465-1477.

Multiple Risk Factor Intervention Trial Research Group. 1990. Mortality rates after 10.5 years for participants in the Multiple Risk Factor Intervention Trial. *Journal of the American Medical Association* 263(13):1795-1801.

Multiple Risk Factor Intervention Trial Research Group. 1996. Mortality after 16 years for participants randomized to the Multiple Risk Factor Intervention Trial. *Circulation* 94(5, Suppl 1):946-951.

Musick MA, Koenig HG, Hays JC, Cohen HJ. 1998. Religious activity and depression among community-dwelling elderly persons with cancer: The moderating effect of race. *Journals of Gerontology Series B Psychological Sciences and Social Sciences* 53(4):S218-S227.

Myers HF, Hwang W-C. 2004. Cumulative psychosocial risks and resilience: A conceptual perspective on ethnic health disparities in late life. In National Research Council, *Critical Perspectives on Racial and Ethnic Differences in Health in Later Life*. Anderson NA, Bulatao RA, Cohen B, eds. Committee on Population, Division of Behavioral and Social Sciences and Education. Washington, DC: The National Academies Press.

Myers HF, Lewis TT, Parker-Dominguez T. 2002. Stress, coping and minority health: Biopsychosocial perspective on ethnic health disparities. In *Handbook of Racial and Ethnic Minority Psychology*. Bernal G, Trimble JE, Burlew AK, Leong FTL, eds. Thousand Oaks, CA: Sage Publications.

Nagashima N, Watanabe T, Nakamura M, Shalabi A, Burdick JF. 2001. Decreased effect of immunosuppression on immunocompetence in African-Americans after kidney and liver transplantation. *Clinical Transplantation* 15(2):111-115.

National Center for Health Statistics. 1994. *Excess Deaths and Other Mortality Measures for the Black Population: 1979-81 and 1991*. Hyattsville, MD: Public Health Service.

National Center for Health Statistics. 2001. *Health, United States, 2001, with Urban and Rural Health Chartbook*. Washington, DC: U.S. Government Printing Office.

National Center for Health Statistics. 2003. *Data Warehouse on Trends in Health and Aging*. Available: http://www.cdc.gov/nchs/agingact.htm [Accessed June 2003].

National Institutes of Health. 1998. *Women of Color Health Data Book: Adolescents to Seniors*. NIH Publication 98-4247. Bethesda, MD: Office of Research on Women's Health, National Institutes of Health.

National Research Council. 1997. *Racial and Ethnic Differences in the Health of Older Americans*. Committee on Population, Martin LG, Soldo BJ, eds. Commission on Behavioral and Social Sciences and Education. Washington, DC: National Academy Press.

National Research Council. 2004. *Critical Perspectives on Racial and Ethnic Differences in Health in Later Life*. Anderson NA, Bulatao RA, Cohen B, eds. Committee on Population, Division of Behavioral and Social Sciences and Education. Washington, DC: The National Academies Press.

Navaie-Waliser M, Feldman PH, Gould DA, Levine C, Kuerbis AN, Donelan K. 2001. The experiences and challenges of informal caregivers: Common themes and differences among whites, black, and hispanics. *Gerontologist* 41(6):733-741.

Nazroo JY. 2004. Ethnic disparities in aging health: What can we learn from the United Kingdom? In National Research Council, *Critical Perspectives on Racial and Ethnic Differences in Health in Later Life*. Anderson NA, Bulatao RA, Cohen B, eds. Committee on Population, Division of Behavioral and Social Sciences and Education. Washington, DC: The National Academies Press.

Neel JV. 1997. Are genetic factors involved in racial and ethnic differences in late-life health? Pp. 210-232 in National Research Council, *Racial and Ethnic Differences in the Health of Older Americans*. Martin LG, Soldo BJ, eds. Committee on Population, Commission on Behavioral and Social Sciences and Education. Washington, DC: National Academy Press.

Neff J. 1984. Race differences in psychological distress: The effects of SES, urbanicity, and measurement strategy. *American Journal of Community Psychology* 12:337-351.

Nei M. 1975. *Molecular Population Genetics and Evolution*. New York: American Elsevier.

Nelson K, Geiger AM, Mangione CM. 2002. Effect of health beliefs on delays in care for abnormal cervical cytology in a multi-ethnic population. *Journal of General Internal Medicine* 17(9):709-716.

Ng B, Dimsdale JE, Rollnik JD, Shapiro H. 1996. The effect of ethnicity on prescriptions for patient-controlled analgesia for post-operative pain. *Pain* 66:9-12.

Nystrom Peck AM. 1992. Childhood environment, intergenerational mobility and adult health: Evidence from Swedish data. *Journal of Epidemiology and Community Health* 46:71-74.

Nystrom Peck AM, Lundberg O. 1995. Short stature as an effect of economic and social conditions in childhood. *Social Science and Medicine* 41(5):733-738.

Nystrom Peck AM, Vagero DH. 1987. Adult body height and childhood socio-economic group in the Swedish population. *Journal of Epidemiology and Community Health* 41.

Oddone EZ, Horner RD, Diers T, Lipscomb J, McIntyre L, Cauffman C, Whittle J, Passman LJ, Kroupa L, Heaney R, Matchar D. 1998. Understanding racial variation in the use of carotid endarterectomy: The role of aversion to surgery. *Journal of the National Medical Association* 90(1):25-33.

Oexmann MJ, Ascanio R, Egan BM. 2001. Efficacy of a church-based intervention on cardiovascular risk reduction. *Ethnicity and Disease* 11(4):817-822.

Office of Management and Budget. 1997. Revisions to the standards for the classification of federal data on race and ethnicity. *Notice* 62(210).

Optenberg SA, Thompson IM, Friedrichs P, Wojcik B, Stein CR, Kramer B. 1995. Race, treatment, and long-term survival from prostate cancer in an equal-access medical care delivery system. *Journal of the American Medical Association* 274(20):1599-1605.

Orth-Gomer K, Eriksson I, Moser V, Theorell T, Fredlund P. 1994. Lipid lowering through work stress reduction. *International Journal of Behavioral Medicine* 1:204-214.

Østbye T, Taylor DH, Jung S-H. 2002. A longitudinal study of the effects of tobacco smoking and other modifiable risk factors on ill health in middle-aged and old Americans: Results from the Health and Retirement Study and Asset and Health Dynamics among the Oldest Old Survey. *Preventive Medicine* 34:334-345.

Otten MW Jr, Teutsch SM, Williamson DF, Marks JS. 1990. The effect of known risk factors on the excess mortality of black adults in the United States. *Journal of the American Medical Association* 263:845-850.

Palloni A, Ewbank DC. 2004. Selection effects in the study of ethnic and race differentials in adult health and mortality. In National Research Council, *Critical Perspectives on Racial and Ethnic Differences in Health in Later Life*. Anderson NA, Bulatao RA, Cohen B, eds. Committee on Population, Division of Behavioral and Social Sciences and Education. Washington, DC: The National Academies Press.

Palloni A, Milesi C. 2002. Social classes, inequalities and health disparities: The intervening role of early health status. Ethnic variations in intergenerational continuities and discontinuities in psychosocial features and disorders. Marbach, Switzerland, October 24-27.

Palloni A, Morenoff JD. 2001. Interpreting the paradoxical in the Hispanic paradox: Demographic and epidemiologic approaches. In *Population Health and Aging: Strengthening the Dialogue Between Epidemiology and Demography.* Weinstein M, Hermalin AI, Stoto MA, eds. Demography and Epidemiology: Frontiers in Population Health and Aging. New York: New York Academy of Sciences.

Pampel FC. 1998. *Aging, Social Inequality, and Public Policy.* Thousand Oaks, CA: Pine Forge Press.

Pearlin LI. 1989. The sociological study of stress. *Journal of Health and Social Behavior* 30:241-256.

Pearlin LI, Wong D, Sexton K. 2001. Residential proximity to industrial sources of air pollution: Interrelationships among race, poverty, and age. *Journal of the Air and Waste Management Association* 51(3):406-421.

Peat JK, Dickerson J, Li J. 1998. Effects of damp and mold in the home on respiratory health: A review of the literature. *Allergy* 53(2):120-128.

Peterson ED, Wright SM, Daley J, Thibault GE. 1994. Racial variation in cardiac procedure use and survival following acute myocardial infarction in the Department of Veterans Affairs. *Journal of the American Medical Association* 271(15):1175-1180.

Peterson ED, Shaw LK, DeLong ER, Pryor DB, Califf RM, Mark DB. 1997. Racial variation in the use of coronary-revascularization procedures: Are the differences real? Do they matter? *New England Journal of Medicine* 36:480-486.

Peto R, Darby S, Deo H, Silcocks P, Whitley E, Doll R. 2000. Smoking, smoking cessation, and lung cancer in the UK since 1950: Combination of national statistics with two case-control studies. *British Medical Journal* 321:323-329.

Pillemer K, Suitor JJ, Landreneau LT, Henderson CR, Brangman S. 2000. Peer support for Alzheimer's caregivers: Lessons from an intervention study. Pp. 265-286 in *Social Integration in the Second Half of Life.* Pillemer K, Moen P, Wethington E, Glasgow N, eds. Baltimore, MD: Johns Hopkins University Press.

Pleis JR, Coles R. 2002. Summary health statistics for U.S. adults: National Health Interview Survey, 1998. *Vital Health Statistics* 10(209).

Polednak AP, King G. 1998. Birth weight of US biracial (black-white) infants: Regional differences. *Ethnicity and Disease* 8:340-349.

Pope CA, Burnett RT, Thun JJ, Calle EE, Krewski D, Ito K, Thurston CD. 2002. Lung cancer, cardiopulmonary mortality, and long-term exposure to fine particulate air pollution. *Journal of the American Medical Association* 287(9):1132-1141.

Powell L. 2002. *Enhancing recovery in coronary heart disease (ENRICHD) trial—Main findings.* Paper presented at the annual meeting of the American Psychosomatic Society, Barcelona, Spain, March.

Power C, Fogelman K, Fox AJ. 1986. Health and social mobility during the early years of life. *Quarterly Journal of Social Affairs* 2(4):397-413.

Power C, Manor O, Fox JA, Fogelman K. 1990. Health in childhood and social inequalities in health in young adults. *Journal of the Royal Statistical Society, Series A* 153(1):17-28.

Power C, Matthews S, Manor O. 1998. Inequalities in self-rated health: Explanations from different stages of life. *Lancet* 351(9108):1009-1014.

Preston SH. 1984. Children and the elderly: Divergent paths for America's dependents. *Demography* 21(4):435-457.

Preston S, Taubman P. 1994. Socioeconomic differences in adult mortality and health status. In National Research Council, *Demography of Aging.* Martin L, Preston S, eds. Committee on Population, Commission on Behavioral and Social Sciences and Education, National Research Council. Washington, DC: National Academy Press.

Preston SH, Hill ME, Drevenstedt GL. 1998. Childhood conditions that predict survival to advanced ages among African-Americans. *Social Science and Medicine* 47(9):1231-1246.

Quadagno J. 2000. Promoting civil rights through the welfare state: How Medicare integrated southern hospitals. *Social Problems* 47:68-89.

Rahkonen O, Lahelma E, Huuhka M. 1997. Past or present? Childhood living conditions and current socioeconomic status as determinants of adult health. *Social Science and Medicine* 44(3):327-336.

Ramsey DJ, Goff DC, Wear ML, Labarthe DR, Nichaman MZ. 1997. Sex and ethnic difference in use of myocardial revascularization procedures in Mexican Americans and non-Hispanic whites: The Corpus Christi Health Project. *Journal of Clinical Epidemiology* 50(5):603-609.

Rathore SS, Lenert LA, Weinfurt KP, Tinoco A, Taleghani CK, Harless W, Schulman KA. 2000. The effects of patient sex and race on medical students' ratings of quality of life. *American Journal of Medicine* 108(7):561-566.

Rathore SS, Foody JM, Wang Y, Smith GL, Herrin J, Masoudi FA, Wolfe P, Havranek EP, Ordin DL, Krumholz HM. 2003. Race, quality of care, and outcomes of elderly patients hospitalized with heart failure. *Journal of the American Medical Association* 289(19):2517-2524.

Raudenbush SW, Sampson RJ. 1999. Ecometrics: Toward a science of assessing ecological settings, with application to the systematic social observation of neighborhoods. *Sociological Methodology* 29(1):1-41.

Rauh VA, Chew GL, Garfinkel RS. 2002. Deteriorating housing contributes to high cockroach allergen levels in inner-city households. *Environmental Health Perspectives* 110:323-327.

Rawls J. 1971. *A Theory of Justice*. Cambridge, MA: Harvard University Press.

Reaven GM. 1988. Banting lecture 1988. Role of insulin resistance in human disease. *Diabetes* 37(12):1595-1607.

Reed DM, Foley DJ, White LR, Heimovitz H, Burchfiel CM, Masaki K. 1998. Predictors of healthy aging in men with high life expectancies. *American Journal of Public Health* 88(10):1463-1468.

Resnicow K, Jackson A, Wang T, De A, McCarty F, Dudley W, Baranowski T. 2001. A motivational interviewing intervention to increase fruit and vegetable intake through black churches: Results of the Eat for Life Trial. *American Journal of Public Health* 91(10):1686-1693.

Risch N, Burchard E, Ziv E, Tang H. 2002. (Opinion) Categorization of humans in biomedical research: Genes, race and disease. *Genome Biology* 3:2007.1-2007.12.

Rodin J, Langer E. 1977. Long-term effects of a control-relevant intervention with the institutionalized aged. *Journal of Personality and Social Psychology* 35:897-902.

Rogers RG, Hummer RA, Nam CB, Peters K. 1996. Demographic, socioeconomic, and behavioral factors affecting ethnic mortality by cause. *Social Forces* 74:1419-1438.

Rogers RG, Hummer RA, Nam CB. 2000. *Living and Dying in the USA*. San Diego, CA: Academic Press.

Rooks RN, Simonsick EM, Miles T, Newman A, Kritchevsky SB, Schulz R, Harris T. 2002. The association of race and socioeconomic status with cardiovascular disease indicators among older adults in the health, aging, and body composition study. *Journal of Gerontology: Social Sciences* 57B(4):S247-S256.

Rosenberg HM, Maurer JD, Sorlie PD, Johnson NJ, MacDorman MF, Hoyert DL, Spitler JF, Scott C. 1999. Quality of death rates by race and Hispanic origin: A summary of current research, 1999. *Vital Health Statistics* 2(128):1-13.

Rosengren A, Orth-Gomer K, Wedel H, Wilhelmsen L. 1993. Stressful life events, social support, and mortality in men born in 1933. *British Medical Journal* 307:1102-1105.

Rosenwaike I. 1987. Mortality differentials among persons born in Cuba, Mexico, and Puerto Rico residing in the United States, 1979-81. *American Journal of Public Health* 77:603-606.

Rössner S. 2001. Obesity in the elderly—A future matter of concern? *Obesity Reviews* 2:183-188.

Roth DL, Haley WE, Owen JE, Clay OJ, Goode KT. 2001. Latent growth models of the longitudinal effects of dementia caregiving: A comparison of African American and white family caregivers. *Psychology and Aging* 16(3):427-436.

Rozanski A, Blumenthal J, Kaplan J. 1999. Impact of psychological factors on the pathogenesis of cardiovascular disease and implications for therapy. *Circulation* 99:2192-2217.

Ruberman W, Weinblatt E, Goldberg JD, Chaudhary BS. 1984. Psychosocial influences on mortality after myocardial infarction. *New England Journal of Medicine* 311(9):552-559.

Rutter M. 1996. Transitions and turning points in developmental psychopathology: As applied to the age span between childhood and mid-adulthood. *International Journal of Behavioral Development* 19:603-626.

Saab P. 2002. *Secondary analyses of psychosocial treatment, demographic and medical variables.* Paper presented at the International Congress of Behavioural Medicine, Helsinki, Finland, August.

Sahota A, Yang M, Gao S, Hui SL, Baiyewu O, Gureje O, Oluwole S, Ogunniyi A, Hall KS, Hendrie HC. 1997. Apolipoprotein E-associated risk for Alzheimer's disease in the African-American population is genotype dependent. *Annals of Neurology* 42:659-661.

Salgado de Snyder VN. 1987. Factors associated with acculturative stress and depressive symptomatology among married Mexican immigrant women. *Psychology of Women Quarterly* 11:475-488.

Sampson RJ, Morenoff JD. 2001. Public health and safety in context: Lessons from community-level theory on social capital. Pp. 366-389 in National Research Council, *Promoting Health: Intervention Strategies from Social and Behavioral Research.* Smedley BD, Syme SL, eds. Washington, DC: National Academy Press.

Sanchez AM, Reed DR, Price RA. 2000. Reduced mortality associated with body mass index (BMI) in African Americans relative to Caucasians. *Ethnicity and Disease* 10:24-30.

Sandefur GD, Campbell ME, Boeck JE. 2004. Racial and ethnic identity, official classifications, and health disparities. In National Research Council, *Critical Perspectives on Racial and Ethnic Differences in Health in Later Life.* Anderson NA, Bulatao RA, Cohen B, eds. Committee on Population, Division of Behavioral and Social Sciences and Education. Washington, DC: The National Academies Press.

Sastry J, Ross CE. 1998. Asian ethnicity and the sense of personal control. *Social Psychology Quarterly* 61(2):101-120.

Satel S. 2000. *PC, M.D.: How Political Correctness Is Corrupting Medicine.* New York: Basic Books.

Satel S. 2001-2002. Medicine's race problem. *Policy Review,* No. 110.

Schnall PL, Landsbergis PA, Baker D. 1994. Job strain and cardiovascular disease. *Annual Review of Public Health* 15:381-411.

Schneider EC, Leape LL, Weissman JS, Piana RN, Gatsonis C, Epstein AM. 2001. Racial differences in cardiac revascularization rates: Does "overuse" explain higher rates among white patients? *Annals of Internal Medicine* 135(5):328-337.

Schoenborn CA, Barnes PM. 2002. Leisure-time physical activity among adults: United States, 1997-98. *Advance Data from Vital and Health Statistics,* No. 325.

Schulman KA, Berlin JA, Harless W, Kerner JF, Sistrunk S, Gersh BJ, Dube R, Taleghani CK, Burke JE, Williams S, Eisenberg J, Escarce JJ, Ayers W. 1999. The effect of race and sex on physicians' recommendations for cardiac catherization. *New England Journal of Medicine* 340:618-626.

Schulz R, Beach SR. 1999. Caregiving as a risk factor for mortality: The Caregiver Health Effects Study. *Journal of the American Medical Association* 282(23):2215-2219.

Schulz R, O'Brien AT, Bookwala J, Fleissner K. 1995. Psychiatric and physical morbidity effects of dementia caregiving: Prevalence, correlates, and causes. *Gerontologist* 35(6):771-791.

Schwartz RS. 2001. Racial profiling in medical research. *New England Journal of Medicine* 344:1392-1393.

Sedlis SP, Fisher VJ, Tice D, Esposito R, Madmon L, Steinberg EH. 1997. Racial differences in performance of invasive cardiac procedures in a Department of Veterans Affairs Medical Center. *Journal of Clinical Epidemiology* 50(8):899-901.

Seeman M, Lewis S. 1997. Powerlessness, health and mortality: A longitudinal study of older men and mature women. *Social Science and Medicine* 41:517-525.

Seeman TE. 1996. Social ties and health. *Annals of Epidemiology* 6:442-451.

Seeman TE, Crimmins E. 2001. Social environment effects on health and aging: Integrating epidemiological and demographic approaches and perspectives. In *Population Health and Aging: Strengthening the Dialogue Between Epidemiology and Demography.* Weinstein M, Hermalin AI, Stoto MA, eds. *Annals of the New York Academy of Sciences* 954:88-117.

Seeman TE, McEwen, BS. 1996. Impact of social environment characteristics on neuroendocrine regulation. *Psychosomatic Medicine* 58:459-471.

Seeman TE, Kaplan GA, Knudsen L, Cohen R, Guralnik J. 1987. Social network ties and mortality among the elderly in the Alameda County Study. *American Journal of Epidemiology* 126:714-723.

Seeman TE, Berkman LF, Kohout F, LaCroix A, Glynn R, Blazer D. 1993. Intercommunity variations in the association between social ties and mortality in the elderly. A comparative analysis of three communities. *Annals of Epidemiology* 3:325-335.

Seeman TE, Charpentier PA, Berkman LF, Tinetti ME, Guralnik JM, Albert M, Blazer D, Rowe JW. 1994. Predicting changes in physical performance in a high-functioning elderly cohort: MacArthur Studies of Successful Aging. *Journal of Gerontology: Medical Sciences* 49(3):M97-M108.

Seeman TE, McAvay G, Merrill S, Albert M, Rodin J. 1996. Self-efficacy beliefs and changes in cognitive performance: MacArthur studies of successful aging. *Psychology and Aging* 11:538-551.

Seeman T, Singer BH, Rowe JW, Horwitz RI, McEwen BS. 1997. Price of adaptation—Allostatic load and its health consequences: MacArthur Studies of Successful Aging. *Archives of Internal Medicine* 157:2259-2268.

Seeman TE, Unger J, McAvay G, Mendes de Leon C. 1999. The role of self-efficacy beliefs in perceptions of functional disability: MacArthur studies of successful aging. *Journal of Gerontology: Psychological Sciences* 54A:P214-P222.

Seeman TE, Lusignolo TM, Albert M, Berkman L. 2001. Social relationships, social support, and patterns of cognitive aging in healthy, high-functioning older adults: MacArthur studies of successful aging. *Health Psychology* 20:243-255.

Seeman TE, Singer B, Ryff C, Levy-Storms L. 2002. Psychosocial factors and the development of allostatic load. *Psychosomatic Medicine* 64:395-406.

Segal SP, Bola RJ, Watson MA. 1996. Race, quality of care, and antipsychotic prescribing practices in psychiatric emergency services. *Psychiatric Services* 47(3):282-286.

Semenza J, Rubin C, Falter K, Selanikio J, Flanders WD, Howe H, Wilhelm J. 1996. Heat-related deaths during the July 1995 heat wave in Chicago. *New England Journal of Medicine* 335:84-90.

Sen A. 2001. Why health equity? Keynote address, International Health Economics Association, York, England, July.

Siegrist J, Peter R, Junge A, Cremer P, Siedel D. 1990. Low status control, high effort at work and ischemic heart disease: Prospective evidence from blue-collar men. *Social Science and Medicine* 31(10):1127-1134.

Simon HA. 1973. The organization of complex systems. In *Hierarchy Theory: The Challenge of Complex Systems*. Pattee HH, ed. New York: George Braziller.

Singer B, Ryff CD. 1999. Hierarchies of life histories and associated health risks. Pp. 96-115 in *Socioeconomic Status and Health in Industrial Nations: Social Psychological, and Biological Pathways*. Adler NE, Marmot M, McEwen BS, Stewart J, eds. New York: New York Academy of Sciences.

Singh GK, Siahpush M. 2002. Ethnic-immigrant differentials in health behaviors, morbidity, and cause-specific mortality in the United States: An analysis of two national data bases. *Human Biology* 74(1):83-109.

Skinner J, Staiger D, Chandra A, Lee J, McClellan M. 2003. Racial differences in hospital quality for the treatment of acute myocardial infarction: Evidence from the Medicare population. Unpublished paper, Dartmouth Medical School.

Smith GD, Kuh D. 1997. Does early nutrition affect later health? Views from the 1930s and 1980s. In *Nutrition in Britain: Science, Scientists and Politics in the Twentieth Century*. Smith DF, ed. London.

Smith JP. 1999. Healthy bodies and thick wallets: The dual relation between health and economic status. *Journal of Economic Perspectives* 13(2):145-166.

Smith JP, Kington RS. 1997. Race, socioeconomic status, and health in late life. Pp. 105-162 in National Research Council, *Racial and Ethnic Differences in the Health of Older Americans*. Martin LG, Soldo BJ, eds. Committee on Population, Commission on Behavioral and Social Sciences and Education. Washington, DC: National Academy Press.

Smith MA, Banjeree S, Gold PW, Glowa J. 1992. Induction of *c-fos* mRNA in rat brain by conditioned and unconditioned stressors. *Brain Research* 578:135-141.

Sondik EJ, Lucas JW, Madans JH, Smith SS. 2000. Race/ethnicity and the 2000 census: Implications for public health. *American Journal of Public Health* 90(11):1709-1713.

Sorlie PD, Backlund E, Johnson NJ, Rogot E. 1993. Mortality by Hispanic status in the United States. *Journal of the American Medical Association* 270:2464-2468.

Splawski I, Timothy KW, Tateyama M, Clancy CE, Malhotra A, Beggs AH, Cappuccio FP, Sagnella GA, Kass RS, Keating MT. 2002. Variant of SCN5A sodium channel implicated in risk of cardiac arrhythmia. *Science* 297:1333.

Steffen PR, Hinderliter AL, Blumenthal JA, Sherwood A. 2001. Religious coping, ethnicity, and ambulatory blood pressure. *Psychosomatic Medicine* 63(4):523-530.

Stern MP, Patterson JK, Mitchell BD, Haffner SM, Hazuda HP. 1990. Overweight and mortality in Mexican Americans. *International Journal of Obesity* 14(7):623-629.

Stevens J. 2000. Obesity and mortality in African-Americans. *Nutrition Reviews* 58(11):346-353.

Stevens J, Kumanyika SK, Keil JE. 1994. Attitudes toward body size and dieting: Differences between elderly black and white women. *American Journal of Public Health* 84:1322-1325.

Stevens J, Cai J, Pamuk ER, Williamson DF, Thun MJ, Wood JL. 1998. The effect of age on the association between body-mass index and mortality. *New England Journal of Medicine* 338(1):1-7.

Stewart AL Verboncoeur DJ, McLellan BY, Gillis DE, Rush S, Mills KM, King AC, Ritter P, White BW, Bortz WM. 2001. Physical activity outcomes of CHAMPS II: A physical activity promotion program for older adults. *Journals of Gerontology Series A: Biological Sciences and Medical Sciences* 56(8):M465-M470.

Strawbridge WJ, Cohen RD, Shema SJ, Kaplan GA. 1996. Successful aging: Predictors and associated activities. *American Journal of Epidemiology* 144(2):135-141.

Strzelczyk JJ, Dignan MB. 2002. Disparities in adherence to recommended followup on screening mammography: Interaction of sociodemographic factors. *Ethnicity and Disease* 12(1):77-86.

Stuck AE, Walthert JM, Nikolaus T, Bula CJ, Hohmann C, Beck JC. 1999. Risk factors for functional status decline in community living elderly people: A systematic literature review. *Social Science and Medicine* 48:445-469.

Sundquist J, Winkleby MA, Pudaric S. 2001. Cardiovascular disease risk factors among older black, Mexican-American, and white women and men: An analysis of NHANES III, 1988-1994. Third National Health and Nutrition Examination Survey. *Journal of the American Geriatrics Society* 49:109-116.

Swallen K. 1997. *Cross-national comparisons of mortality differentials: Immigrants to the US and stayers in common countries of origin.* Paper presented at the annual meetings of the Population Association of America, Washington, DC, March.

Syme SL. 2002. *Interventions to reduce health disparities: Should they be specifically targeted or universally applicable?* Paper prepared for the Panel on Race, Ethnicity, and Health in Later Life. Washington, DC: National Research Council.

Taioli E, Crofts F, Trachman J, Bayo S, Toniolo P, Garte SJ. 1995. Racial differences in CYP1A1 genotype and function. *Toxicology Letters* 77:357-362.

Taylor AJ, Meyer GS, Morse RW, Pearson CE. 1997. Can characteristics of a health care system mitigate ethnic bias in access to cardiovascular procedures? Experience from the military health services system. *Journal of the American College of Cardiology* 30:901-907.

Taylor CB, Bandura A, Ewart CK, Miller NH, Debusk RF. 1985. Raising spouse's and patient's perception of his cardiac capabilities after clinically uncomplicated acute myocardial function. *American Journal of Cardiology* 55:635-638.

Taylor RJ, Chatters LM. 1988. Church members as a source of informal social support. *Review of Religious Research* 30:193-203.

Thayer JF, Friedman BH. 2004. A neurovisceral integration model of health disparities in aging. In National Research Council, *Critical Perspectives on Racial and Ethnic Differences in Health in Later Life.* Anderson NA, Bulatao RA, Cohen B, eds. Committee on Population, Division of Behavioral and Social Sciences and Education. Washington, DC: The National Academies Press.

Theorell R, Emdad R, Arnetz B, Weingarten A-M. 2001. Employee effects of an educational program for managers at an insurance company. *Psychosomatic Medicine* 63:724-733.

Theorell T, Tsutsumi A, Hallquist J. 1998. Decision latitude, job strain, and myocardial infarction: A study of working men in Stockholm. *American Journal of Public Health* 88(3):382-388.

Thompson VLS. 1996. Perceived experiences of racism as stressful life events. *Community Mental Health Journal* 32:223-233.

Thun MJ, Peto R, Lopez AD, Monaco JH, Henley SJ, Heath CW Jr, Doll R. 1997. Alcohol consumption and mortality among middle-aged and elderly U.S. adults. *New England Journal of Medicine* 337(24):1705-1714.

Thurlbeck WM. 1992. Prematurity and the developing lung. *Clinical Perinatology* 19:497-519.

Thurston GD, Ito K. 2001. Epidemiological studies of acute ozone exposures and mortality. *Journal of Exposure Analysis and Environmental Epidemiology* 11(4):286-294.

Todd KH, Samaroo N, Hoffman JR. 1993. Ethnicity as a risk factor for inadequate emergency department analgesia. *Journal of the American Medical Association* 269:1537-1539.

Todd KH, Deaton C, D'Adamo AP, Goe L. 2000. Ethnicity and analgesia practice. *Annals of Emergency Medicine* 35(1):11-16.

Torsch VL, Ma GX. 2000. Cross-cultural comparison of health perceptions, concerns, and coping strategies among Asian and Pacific Islander American elders. *Qualitative Health Research* 10(4):471-489.

Troxel WM, Matthews KA, Bromberger JT, Sutton-Tyrrell K. 2003. Chronic stress burden, discrimination, and subclinical carotid artery disease in African American and Caucasian women. *Health Psychology* 22(3):300-309.

Turner JR, Sherwood A, Light KC. 1992. *Individual Differences in Cardiovascular Responses to Stress.* New York: Plenum.

Turvey C, Wallace R, Herzog R. 1999. A revised CES-D measure of depressive symptoms and a DSM-based measure of major depressive episodes in the elderly. *International Psychogeriatrics* 11:139-148.

U.S. Census Bureau. 1990. Characteristics of American Indians by tribe and language: 1990 Census of Population (1990 CP-3-7). Available: http://www.census.gov/population/www/socdemo/race/cp-3-7.html [Accessed March 2003].

U.S. Census Bureau. 2001. Current Population Survey, March 2000. Available: http://www.census.gov/population/socdemo/foreign/p20-534/tab0301.txt [Accessed March 2003].

U.S. Census Bureau. 2002a. Annual projections of the resident population by age, sex, race, and Hispanic origin: Lowest, middle, highest, and zero international migration series, 1999 to 2100. Available: http://www.census.gov/population/www/projections/natdet.html [Accessed December 2002].

U.S. Census Bureau. 2002b. Modified race data summary file, 2000 Census of Population and Housing, Technical documentation. Available: eire.census.gov/popest/data/national/tables/files/mod_race.php#abs [Accessed December 2002].

U.S. Department of Health and Human Services. 1998. *Tobacco Use among U.S. Racial/ Ethnic Minority Groups—African Americans, American Indian and Alaska Natives, Asian Americans and Pacific Islanders, and Hispanics: A Report of the Surgeon General.* Atlanta: U.S. Department of Health and Human Services, Centers for Disease Control and Prevention, National Center for Chronic Disease Prevention and Health Promotion, Office on Smoking and Health.

U.S. Department of Health and Human Services. 2000. *Reducing Tobacco Use: A Report of the Surgeon General.* Atlanta: U.S. Department of Health and Human Services, Centers for Disease Control and Prevention, National Center for Chronic Disease Prevention and Health Promotion, Office on Smoking and Health.

U.S. Department of Health, Education, and Welfare. 1964. *Smoking and Health: Report of the Advisory Committee to the Surgeon General of the Public Health Service.* Washington, DC: U.S. Department of Health Education, and Welfare. Public Health Service.

U.S. Department of Health, Education, and Welfare. 1979. *Healthy People: The Surgeon General's Report on Health Promotion and Disease Prevention.* DHEW Pub. No. (PHS) 79-55071. Washington, DC: U.S. Government Printing Office.

Uchino BN, Cacioppo JT, Keicolt-Glaser JK. 1996. The relationship between social support and physiological processes: A review with emphasis on underlying mechanisms and implications for health. *Psychological Bulletin* 119(3):488-531.

Ulbrich P, Warheit G, Zimmerman R. 1989. Race, socioeconomic status, and psychological distress: An examinatin of differential vulnerability. *Journal of Health and Social Behavior* 30:131-146.

Uppaluri CR, Schumm LP, Lauderdale DS. 2001. Self-reports of stress in Asian immigrants: Effects of ethnicity and acculturation. *Ethnicity and Disease* 11(1):107-114.

Utsey SO, Ponterotto JG. 1996. Development and validation of the index of race-related stress (IRRS). *Journal of Consulting Psychology* 43(4):490-501.

Vagero D, Leon D. 1994. Ischaemic heart disease and low birth weight: A test of the fetal-origins hypothesis from the Swedish twin registry. *Lancet* 343.

Vague P, Raccah D. 1992. The syndrome of insulin resistance. *Hormone Research* 38(1-2):28-32.

Van den Berghe P. 1964. *Race and Racism: A Comparative Perspective.* New York: Wiley.

van Ryn M. 2002. Research on the provider contribution to race/ethnicity disparities in medical care. *Medical Care* 40(1):I140-I151.

van Ryn M, Burke J. 2000. The effect of patient race and socio-economic status on physician's perceptions of patients. *Social Science and Medicine* 50:813-828.

van Ryn M, Fu SS. 2003. Paved with good intentions: Do public health and human service providers contribute to racial/ethnic disparities in health? *American Journal of Public Health* 93(2):248-255.

van Ryn M, Hannan E, Burke J, Besculides M. 1999. *An Examination of Factors Associated with Physician Recommendations for Revascularization.* Washington, DC: American Public Health Association.

Vaupel JW, Yashin AI. 1985. Heterogeneity's ruses: Some surprising effects of selection on population dynamics. *American Statistician* 39(3):176-185.

Vaupel J, Manton K, Stallard E. 1979. The impact of heterogeneity in individual frailty on the dynamics of mortality. *Demography* 16(3):439-554.

Vieira C, Pasyukova EG, Zeng Z-B, Hackett JB, Lyman RF, Mackay TFC. 2000. Genotype-environment interaction for quantitative trait loci affecting life span in *Drosophila melanogaster. Genetics* 154:213-227.

Vitaliano P, Schulz R, Kiecolt-Glaser J, Grant I. 1997. Research on physiological and physical concomitants of caregiving: Where do we go from here? *Annals of Behavioral Medicine* 19:117-123.

Vitaliano PP, Scanlan JM, Zhang J, Savage MV, Hirsch IB, Siegler IC. 2002. A path model of chronic stress, The metabolic syndrome, and coronary heart disease. *Psychosomatic Medicine* 64(3):418-435.

Waddington CH. 1977. *Tools for Thought.* New York: Basic Books.

Wadsworth MEJ. 1986. Serious illness in childhood and its association with later-life achievement. In *Class and Health.* New York: Tavistock Publications.

Wadsworth MEJ. 1991. *The Imprint of Time: Childhood, History and Adult Life.* Oxford: Clarendon Press.

Wadsworth MEJ, Kuh DJL. 1997. Childhood influences on adult health: A review of recent work from the British 1946 National Birth Cohort Study, the MRC National Survey of Health and Development. *Paediatric and Perinatal Epidemiology* 11:2-20.

Waidmann TA, Rajan S. 2000. Race and ethnic disparities in health care access and utilization: An examination of state variation. *Medical Care Research and Review* 57(Suppl 1):55-84.

Wallace SP, Enriquez-Haass V, Markides K. 1998. The consequences of color-blinding health policy for older racial and ethnic minorities. *Stanford Law and Policy Review* 9(2):329-346.

Warheit GJ, Holzer CE 3rd, Schwab JJ. 1973. An analysis of social class and racial differences in depressive symptomatology: A community study. *Journal of Health and Social Behavior* 14(4):291-299.

Warheit GJ, Holzer CE 3rd, Arey SA. 1975. Race and mental illness: An epidemiologic update. *Journal of Health and Social Behavior* 16(3):243-256.

Warner DF, Hayward MD. 2002. *Race disparities in men's mortality: The role of childhood social conditions in a process of cumulative disadvantage.* Paper presented at the annual meetings of the Population Association of America, Atlanta, May 9-11.

Warner KE. 2001. The need for, and value of, a multi-level approach to disease prevention: The case of tobacco control. In National Research Council, *Promoting Health: Intervention Strategies from Social and Behavioral Research.* Smedley BD, Syme SL, eds. Washington, DC: National Academy Press.

Waters MC. 2000. Immigration, intermarriage, and the challenge of measuring racial/ethnic identities. *American Journal of Public Health* 90:1735-1737.

Weinick RM, Zuvekas SH, Cohen JW. 2000. Racial and ethnic differences in access to and use of health care services. 1977 to 1996. *Medical Care Research Review* 57 (Suppl 1):36-54.

Weisse CS, Sorum PC, Sanders KN, Syat BL. 2001. Do gender and race affect decisions about pain management? *Journal of General Internal Medicine* 16(4):211-217.

Weitz JS, Fraser HB. 2001. Explaining mortality rate plateaus. *Proceedings of the National Academy of Sciences* 98(26):15383-15386.

Wennberg JE, Cooper M, eds. 1999. *Dartmouth Atlas of Health Care 1999.* Chicago: Dartmouth Medical School and American Hospital Association.

West P. 1991. Rethinking the health selection explanation for health inequalities. *Social Science and Medicine* 32(4):373-384.

White IR, Altmann DR, Nanchahal K. 2002. Alcohol consumption and mortality: Modelling risks for men and women at different ages. *British Medical Journal* 325:191.

White TN, Williams DR, Jackson JS, et al. 2000. Being black and feeling blue: The mental health consequences of racial discrimination. *Race and Society* 2:117-131.

Whiteley K, Hurwitz B, Schneiderman N. 1999. Ethnic variations in the pharmacological and nonpharmacological treatment of hypertension: Biopsychosocial perspective. *Human Biology* 71(4):607-639.

Whitman S, Good G, Donoghue ER, Benbow N, Shou W, Mou S. 1997. Mortality in Chicago attributed to the July 1995 heat wave. *American Journal of Public Health* 87(9):1515-1518.

Whittemore AS. 1989. Colorectal cancer incidence among Chinese in North America and the People's Republic of China: Variation with sex, age, and anatomical site. *International Journal of Epidemiology* 18(3):563-568.

Whittle J, Conigliaro J, Good CB, Lofgren RP. 1993. Racial differences in the use of invasive cardiovascular procedures in the Department of Veterans Affairs Medical System. *New England Journal of Medicine* 329(9):621-627.

Wilkinson RG. 1997. *Unhealthy Societies: The Afflictions of Inequality.* London: Routledge.

Williams DR. 1990. Socioeconomic differentials in health: A review and redirection. *Social Psychology Quarterly* 53(2):81-99.

Williams DR. 2000. Race, stress, and mental health: Findings from the Commonwealth Minority Health Survey. Pp. 209-243 in *Minority Health in America: Findings and Policy Implications from the Commonwealth Fund Minority Health Survey.* Hogue C, Hargraves M, Scott-Collins K, eds. Baltimore, MD: Johns Hopkins University Press.

Williams DR. 2001a. Race and health: Trends and policy implications. Pp. 67-85 in *Income, Socioeconomic Status, and Health: Exploring the Relationships*. Auerbach JA, Krimgold BK, eds. Washington, DC: National Policy Association, Academy for Health Services Research and Health Policy.

Williams DR. 2001b. Racial variations in adult health status: Patterns, paradoxes, and prospects. Pp. 371-410 in *America Becoming: Racial Trends and Their Consequences*, Vol. 2. Smelser NJ, Wilson WJ, Mitchell F, eds. Washington, DC: National Academy Press.

Williams DR, Collins C. 1995. U.S. socioeconomic and racial differences in health: Patterns and explanations. *Annual Review of Sociology* 21:349-386.

Williams DR, Collins CA. 2001. Racial residential segregation: A fundamental cause of racial disparities in health. *Public Health Reports* 116:404-415.

Williams DR, Neighbors HW. 2001. Racism, discrimination and hypertension: Evidence and needed research. *Ethnicity and Disease* 11(Suppl):800-816.

Williams D, Wilson C. 2001. Race, ethnicity, and aging. Pp. 160-178 in *Handbook of Aging and the Social Sciences*, 5th ed. Binstock RH, George LK, eds. San Diego: Academic Press.

Williams DR, HW Neighbors, JS Jackson. 2003. Racial/ethnic discrimination and health: Findings from community studies. *American Journal of Public Health* 93(2):200-208.

Williams RB, Barefoot JC, Califf RM, Haney TL, Saunders WB, Pryor DB, Hlatky MA, Siegler IC, Mark DB. 1992. Prognostic importance of social and economic resources among medically treated patients with angiographically documented coronary artery disease. *Journal of the American Medical Association* 267:520-524.

Williams SW, Dilworth-Anderson P. 2002. Systems of social support in families who care for dependent African American elders. *Gerontologist* 42(2):224-236.

Wilson JF, Weale ME, Smith AC, Gratrix G, Fletcher B, Thomas MG, Bradman N, Goldstein DB. 2001. Population genetic structure of variable drug response. *Nature Genetics* 29:265-269.

Winkleby MA, Cubbin C. 2004. Racial/ethnic disparities in health behaviors: A challenge to current assumptions. In National Research Council, *Critical Perspectives on Racial and Ethnic Differences in Health in Later Life*. Anderson NA, Bulatao RA, Cohen B, eds. Committee on Population, Division of Behavioral and Social Sciences and Education. Washington, DC: The National Academies Press.

Wong MD, Shapiro MF, Boscardin WJ, Ettner SL. 2002. Contribution of major diseases to disparities in mortality. *New England Journal of Medicine* 347(20):1585-1592.

World Health Organization. 2002. *The World Health Report 2002: Reducing Risks, Promoting Healthy Life*. Geneva: World Health Organization.

Yancey WL, Ericksen EP, Juliani RN. 1976. Emergent ethnicity: A review and reformulation. *American Sociological Review* 41(3):391-403.

Yanek LR, Becker DM, Moy TF, Gittelsohn J, Koffman DM. 2001. Project Joy: Faith based cardiovascular health promotion for African American women. *Public Health Reports* 116(Suppl 1):68-81.

Yashin AI, De Benedictis G, Vaupel JW, Tan Q, Andreev KF, Iachine IA, Bonafe M, DeLuca M, Valensin S, Carotenuto L, Franceschi C. 1999. Genes, demography, and life span: The contribution of demographic data in genetic studies on aging and longevity. *American Journal of Human Genetics* 65(4):1178-1193.

Zambrana RE, Scrimshaw SC, Collins N, Dunkel-Shetter C. 1997. Prenatal health behaviors and psychological risk factors in pregnant women of Mexican origin: The role of acculturation. *American Journal of Public Health* 87(6):1022-1026.

Ziegler RG, Hoover RN, Pike MD, Hildesheim A, Nomura AMY, West DW, Wu-Williams AH, Kolonal LN, Horn-Ross PL, Rosenthal JF, Hyer MB. 1993. Migration patterns and breast cancer risk in Asian American women. *Journal of the National Cancer Institute* 85:1819-1826.
Zoratti R. 1998. A review on ethnic differences in plasma triglycerides and high-density-lipoprotein cholesterol: Is the lipid pattern the key factor for the low coronary heart disease rate in people of African origin? *European Journal of Epidemiology* 14(1):9-21.

Appendix

Contents,
Critical Perspectives on Racial and Ethnic Differences in Health in Late Life

The papers in *Critical Perspectives on Racial and Ethnic Differences in Health in Late Life* (National Research Council, 2004) were originally presented in March 2002 at the Panel's Workshop on Ethnic Disparities in Aging. They were subsequently modified to incorporate the comments of discussants at the workshop, panel members, and reviewers. The papers and the workshop discussion contributed significantly to the panel's work and this report.

Biographical Sketches

NORMAN B. ANDERSON (*Chair*) is professor of health and social behavior at Harvard University. His research interests involve ethnic, racial, and socioeconomic disparities in health; the social, behavioral, and biological processes underlying them; and interventions to reduce such disparities. Until recently, Dr. Anderson was director of the Office of Behavioral and Social Sciences Research at the National Institutes of Health (NIH). As the founding director of that office, he worked to promote and set priorities in behavioral and social science research and training throughout NIH, oversaw a tripling of the operating budget of the office, and organized funding initiatives totaling $90 million over 4 years. Dr. Anderson was previously at Duke University, where he studied the role of stress in the development of hypertension and directed the NIH-funded Exploratory Center for Research on Health Promotion in Older Minorities. He is a fellow of the American Psychological Association, the American Psychological Society, the Society of Behavioral Medicine, and the Academy of Behavioral Medicine Research and past president of the Society of Behavioral Medicine. He has a Ph.D. in psychology from the University of North Carolina at Greensboro, with postdoctoral training in aging and psychophysiology from Duke University.

RODOLFO A. BULATAO served as staff director for most of the panel's life. His research has covered psychosocial issues in population, fertility determinants, family planning program effectiveness, and program and reproductive health service costs. He previously directed the World Bank's annual population projections and has worked on projections in various areas, including causes of death. He has also helped develop and evaluate population projects in developing countries. Dr. Bulatao was previously affiliated with the East-West Center and the University of the Philippines. He served on the staff of the National Research Council's Committee on Population in 1983-1985 and with its Working Group on Population Growth and Economic Development. He has an M.A. in sociology from the University of the Philippines and a Ph.D. in sociology from the University of Chicago.

EILEEN M. CRIMMINS is the Edna M. Jones professor of gerontology and sociology at the University of Southern California and director of the USC/UCLA Center for Biodemography and Population Health. Her work has concentrated on trends and differentials in population health. She has also worked to develop measures of healthy life as indicators for assessing population health trends and differentials. Her current work is on the role of biological factors in explaining racial/ethnic, educational, and income differentials in health. She has a Ph.D. in demography from the University of Pennsylvania.

DAVID V. ESPINO is a professor of family medicine and geriatrics and Vice Chair for Community Geriatrics in the Department of Family and Community Medicine at the University of Texas Health Science Center at San Antonio. He has authored over 100 publications dealing with clinical issues of Mexican American elders, and he serves as the director of the John A. Hartford Center of Geriatric Excellence, one of 23 such centers nationally. Dr. Espino is also a member of the National Advisory Council of the National Institute on Aging and a fellow of the American Academy of Family Physicians and the American Geriatrics Society. He is a graduate of the University of Texas Medical Branch at Galveston and completed a family medicine residency at Spohn-Memorial Medical Center in Corpus Christi and a geriatrics fellowship at Mount Sinai Medical Center in New York City and holds a certificate of added qualifications in geriatrics.

JAMES S. HOUSE is director of the Survey Research Center, professor in the Department of Sociology, and research scientist in the Survey Research Center of the Institute of Social Research and the Department of Epidemiology, all at the University of Michigan. His research has spanned such areas as social psychology, social structure and personality, psychosocial and socioeconomic factors in health and aging, survey research methods, and political sociology. Among his numerous publications are recent articles on understanding and reducing socioeconomic and racial/ethnic disparities in health; income inequality and mortality; socioeconomic inequalities in health; and gender and the socioeconomic gradient in mortality. Dr. House is a member of the Institute of Medicine and a recipient of the Robert Wood

Johnson Foundation Investigator Awards in Health Policy Research. He has a Ph.D. in social psychology from the University of Michigan.

JAMES S. JACKSON is the Daniel Katz distinguished university professor of psychology and professor of health behavior and health education at the University of Michigan. He is also director of the Center for Afro-American and African Studies and director of the Research Center for Group Dynamics, Institute for Social Research, where he also directs the Program for Research on Black Americans, now in its 25th year. He has published numerous scientific articles and chapters in such areas as race and ethnic relations, health and mental health, adult development and aging, attitudes and attitude change, and black political behavior, and he has authored or coauthored several books and edited volumes. Dr. Jackson has chaired the Gerontological Society Task Force on Racial Minority Group Aging and is a past chair of the Behavioral and Social Science Section of the Gerontological Society of America. He has been a member of scientific review panels for such organizations as the National Institute of Mental Health, the National Cancer Institute, the Educational Testing Service, and the European Economic Community Study on Immigration and Racism. He is a past member of national advisory councils of the National Institute of Mental Health and the National Institute on Aging (NIA). He currently serves as a member of the NIA's Board of Scientific Counselors and also chaired a recent panel on minority aging at the NIA. He received a Ph.D. in social psychology from Wayne State University.

CHRISTOPHER (SANDY) JENCKS is Malcolm Wiener professor of social policy at the Kennedy School at Harvard University. His recent research has dealt with changes in the material standard of living over the past generation, homelessness, welfare reform, the black-white test score gap, and poverty measurement. His books have covered inequality, the urban underclass, and the homeless. Dr. Jencks is a member of the National Academy of Sciences and the American Academy of Arts and Sciences, and he serves on the editorial board of *The American Prospect.*

GERALD E. MCCLEARN is Evan Pugh professor and director of the Center for Development and Health Genetics in the College of Health and Human Development at Pennsylvania State University. Previously, he taught at Yale University, Allegheny College, the University of California at Berkeley, and the University of Colorado. At the University of Colorado he founded the Institute for Behavioral Genetics. Subsequently at Pennsylvania State University he served as associate dean for research and dean of the College of Health and Human Development. He was the founding head of the program in biobehavioral health and founding director of the Center for Development and Health Genetics. He has been involved for the past

15 years in large-scale studies of genetic and environmental influences on patterns and rates of aging in Swedish twins. He has been president of the Behavioral Genetics Association and he received a MERIT award from the National Institute on Aging in 1994. He holds a Ph.D. from the University of Wisconsin.

ALBERTO PALLONI is professor of demography at the Center for Demography and Ecology and in the Departments of Sociology and Preventive Medicine at the University of Wisconsin-Madison. His primary research interests are the demography of health and mortality, population dynamics in developing countries, and demography of HIV/AIDS in Africa. He also works on mathematical demography and statistical methods. His works include papers on the demography of HIV/AIDS, the effects of economic crises on fertility and mortality, and research on socioeconomic determinants of health and mortality. He currently serves on the National Research Council's Committee on Population and previously served on the Panel on Decennial Census Methodology. He has a Ph.D. in sociology from the University of Washington.

TERESA SEEMAN is professor of medicine and epidemiology in the Schools of Medicine and of Public Health at the University of California at Los Angeles. Her research focuses on the role in health and aging of sociocultural factors, specifically on the biological pathways involved. Recent publications have covered allostatic load and its health consequences, the effects of the social environment on neuroendocrine function, and how an unhealthy environment "gets under the skin." Dr. Seeman was a member of the MacArthur Research Network on Successful Aging (1985-1995) and is currently a member of the MacArthur Research Network on Socioeconomic Status and Health. She was previously on the faculty of the Department of Epidemiology in the Yale School of Public Health and at the Andrus School of Gerontology at the University of Southern California. She received a Ph.D. in epidemiology from the University of California at Berkeley.

JAMES P. SMITH is the RAND chair in labor markets and demographic studies; previously, he directed RAND's Labor and Population Studies Program. He has been closely involved since their inception in the design and operation of both the Health and Retirement Survey (HRS) and Asset and Health Dynamics of the Oldest-Old (AHEAD). As chair of an advisory panel of the National Institute on Aging (NIA) extramural priorities for data collection in health and retirement economics, he authored a report outlining the thematic design for these new surveys and calling for NIA support. Subsequently, he served on the NIA Data Monitoring Committee for both surveys. He has written a number of papers on the quality of asset data in both HRS and AHEAD and racial and ethnic differences in personal net worth, Social Security, and pension wealth. Dr. Smith is also a member of the National Science Foundation Advisory Committee for the Panel Study of Income Dynamics and is the public representative appointed by the governor of California on the state board for the Occupational Safety and Health Administration. He has served on the National Advisory Board for the Poverty Institute and on the Population Research Committee at the National Institutes of Health. He has received the National Institutes of Health MERIT Award. He has a Ph.D. in economics from the University of Chicago.

EUGENIA WANG is professor of biochemistry and molecular biology in the School of Medicine at the University of Louisville. Previously, she was professor of anatomy and cell biology and of neurology and neurosurgery at McGill University in Montréal, where she was also director of the Bloomfield Center for Research in Aging at the Lady Davis Institute for Medical Research. Dr. Wang has investigated the molecular mechanisms controlling the process of aging, at both cellular and organismic levels. Her recent work involves the investigation of gene-directed programs regulating the ontogeny of age-dependent diseases, and how genetic action in individual cells controls human longevity, integrating microarray technology, mathematical genomics, and pattern recognition theory to identify genetic and epigenetic factors as life-span determinants. She is chair of the biological science section of the Gerontological Society of America and has served as chair of the biological science section of the Canadian Association on Gerontology. She was also a member of the Minority Aging Ad Hoc Review Committee for the National Advisory Council on Aging. Dr. Wang received her B.S. from the National Taiwan University, her M.Sc. from Northern Michigan University, and her Ph.D. from Case Western Reserve University.

DAVID R. WILLIAMS is professor of sociology and senior research scientist at the Institute for Social Research at the University of Michigan. His prior academic appointment was at Yale University. Dr. Williams is interested in social and psychological factors that affect health and especially in the trends and the determinants of socioeconomic and racial differences in mental and physical health. Currently, he is on the editorial board of five scientific journals. He also served on the Department of Health and Human Services National Committee on Vital and Health Statistics, chairing its subcommittee on minority and other special populations. He has held such elected positions in professional organizations as secretary-treasurer of the Medical Sociology Section of the American Sociological Association. He received an M.P.H. from Loma Linda University and a Ph.D. in sociology from the University of Michigan.

Index

A

Access to health care, 3, 7, 36, 92, 93
 see also Health insurance; Patient
  compliance; Self-care practices;
  Utilization of health care
 early life disadvantage, 107
 prejudice and discrimination, 77
 research recommendations, 6, 102
Adolescents
 multiracial self-identification, 10
 National Longitudinal Survey of Youth,
  108
 socioeconomic status and behavior risk
  factors, 35
African Americans, *see* Black persons
Age factors, *see* Life cycle factors
AIDS, *see* HIV
Alaska Natives, 1
 behavioral risk factors, 62, 63, 68
 health and disability, general, 20-21, 26,
  29
 health insurance, 95
 historical perspectives, 12
 mortality, 17, 26
 prejudice and discrimination, 81
 quality of health care, 97
 racial/ethnic identification, 9, 10-11, 13,
  14

research recommendations, 26, 28
 reservation inhabitants, 13-14
 risk factors, 28
 socioeconomic status, 56-57
Alcohol use and abuse, 32, 61, 62, 63, 64, 66
 prejudice and discrimination, 78
Alternative and complementary medicine,
  112
 research recommendations, 6, 114
Alzheimer's disease and dementia, 20, 23
 genetics and, 50
 psychosocial factors, 72
 stress on spouse, 83
American Indians, 1
 see also Alaska Natives
 behavioral risk factors, 62, 63, 68, 118
 causes of death, 18, 19
 health and disability, general, 20-21, 26,
  29
 health insurance, 95
 health promotion, 113
 hospitalization, 13-14
 mortality, 13, 16, 17, 18, 26
 prejudice and discrimination, 12, 81
 quality of health care, 96, 97
 racial/ethnic identification, 9, 10, 11, 13-
  14
 research recommendations, 26, 28
 reservation inhabitants, 13-14, 29